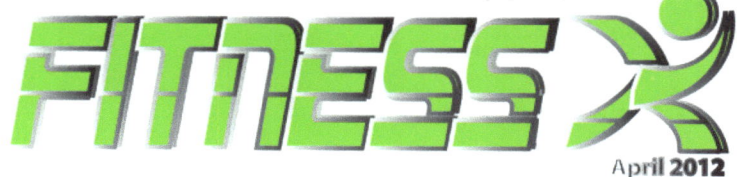

April **2012**

KERI LYNN FORD

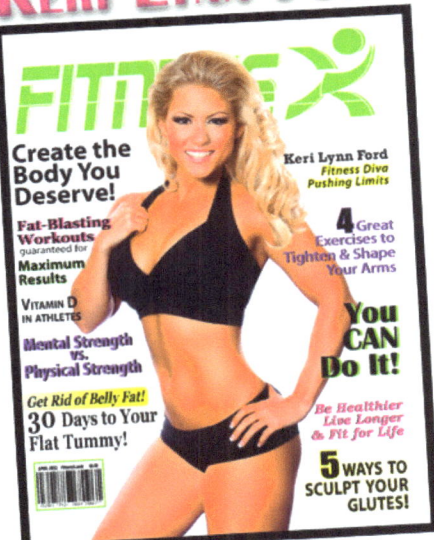

You will get full access to all articles on
Health, Wellness, Nutrition, Healthy Recipes,
Training, Exercise Routines, Transformations, Events,
Inspirational Stories, Champions of Fitness,
Fit Model of the Month, &
Full-Page Photos of our Inspiring
Professional Fitness Models and Athletes!
All of this with very few advertisements!

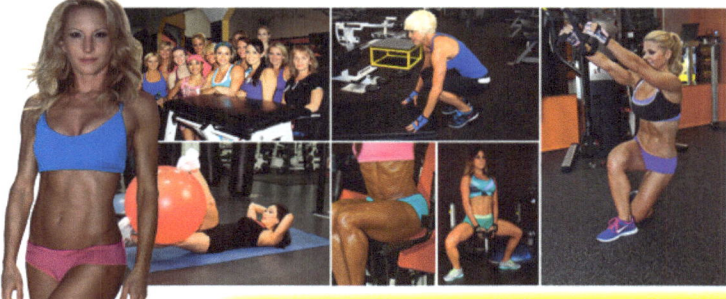

Get all **5 WORKOUTS**
to target <u>every</u> body part &
**ACHIEVE THE RESULTS
YOU WANT!**

Purchase *FitnessX Magazine!*

**Digital on Kindle, iPad, iPhone & Android & Print
Go to Amazon.com & type FitnessX Magazine in the search box!**

FitnessX Magazine
hopes to inspire and motivate women
to live a healthy lifestyle.
Our writers/models will inspire you
with articles as well as tips
about fitness, health and wellness.
All our models are natural athletes
and excel in other disciplines.

At *FitnessX Magazine*, our tagline says it all--
"Inspiring You to Live Well...Naturally!"

It's
NOW you can READ
FitnessX Magazine
on your iPad, iPhone,
Android & Kindle Fire!
Download the Kindle app
to your device!

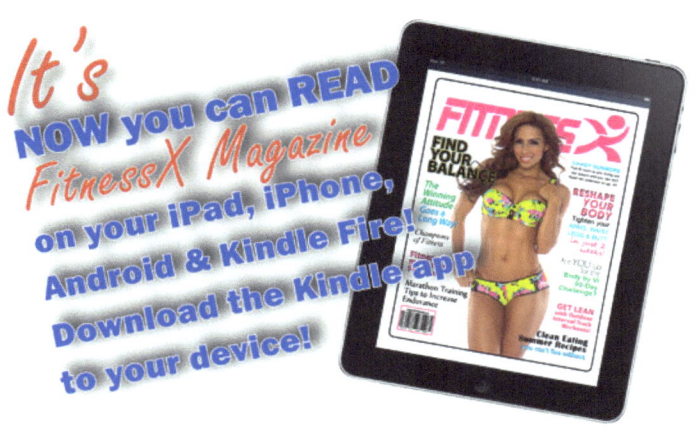

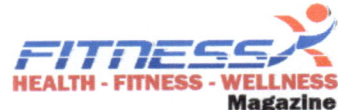

HEALTH

20. VITAMIN D FOR ATHLETES

27. ASK THE DENTIST - WATER FLUORIDATION

NUTRITION

8. THE NAKED TRUTH

17. HEALTHY RESULTS WITH APPLE CIDER VINEGAR

29. HOW TO EAT LESS & ENJOY MORE

EXERCISE

12. NICOLE'S GLUTE BUSTING WORKOUT

14. GET TANK TOP READY-ARM WORKOUT

22. WELCOME BACK ABS

WELLNESS

8. GET YOUR MIND RIGHT

27. HAPPINESS LIES WITHIN

TRAINING

3. BIKRAM YOGA & COMPETITIVE FITNESS

32. 6 STEPS TO YOUR 6-PACK

OTHER CONTENT

11. LEHA LONG'S -COMPETITOR'S CORNER!

24. WHAT FOREVER CHANGED ME

28. I AM A COMPETITOR, A SURVIVOR

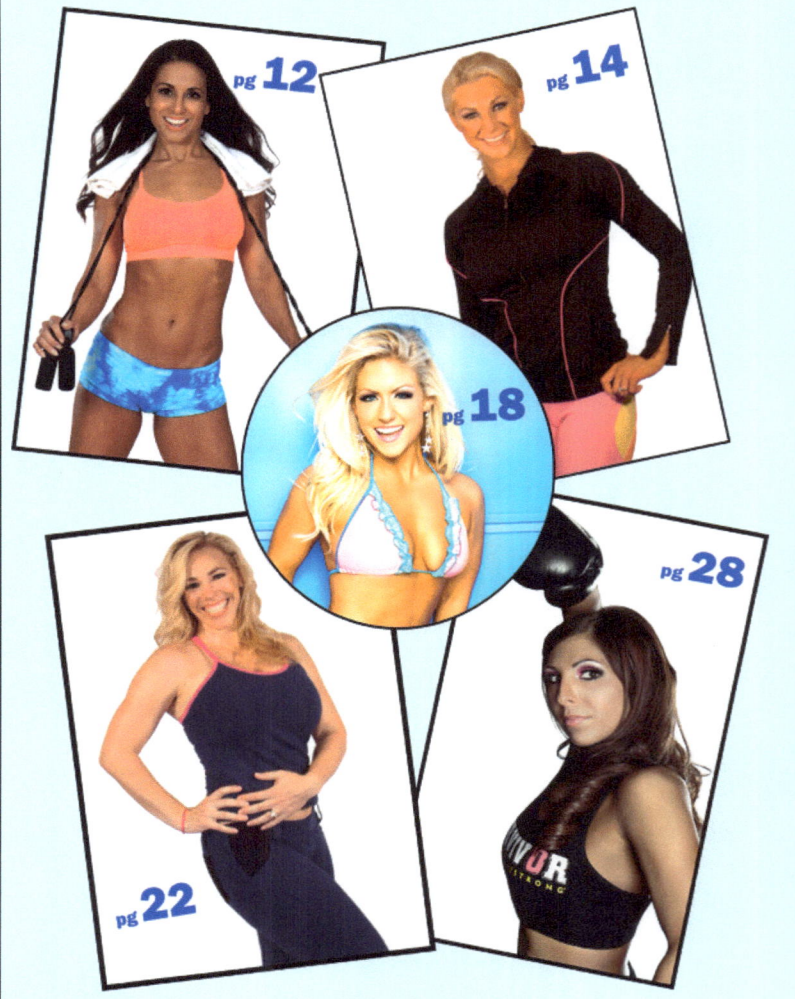

pg 12

pg 14

pg 18

pg 28

pg 22

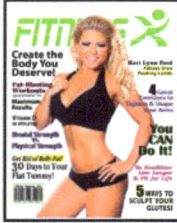

APRIL 2012 COVER
Cover Model:
KERI LYNN FORD

Cover Photographer:
EVA SIMON PHOTOGRAPHY

SITES:
fitnessX.com
twitter.com/fitnessX
youtube.com/fitnessXtv
facebook.com/fitnessXmag
fitnessxisbodyproud.com

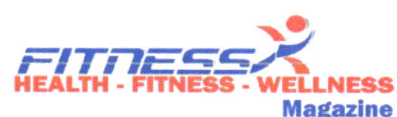

APRIL 2012

Publishers:
Kat Painter and BillyBow

Editor-in-Chief
Kat Painter

Assistant Editor/Copy Editor
April Branton

Pregnancy Fitness Specialist:
Laura Mak Quist

Creative Director:
Kat Painter and BillyBow

Senior Designer:
Kat Painter and Taylor Anne Kinkade

Senior Staff Photographers:
B-House Photography and Natalie Lynn Lichtenbert

Photographers:
BillyBow Photography, B-House Photography, Eva Simon Photography, PictureGroove Photography, Noel Daganta, James Patrick Photography, Excipio Photograf, Bersano Photography, Nicholson Studios, Jesus Esquivel, Raw Images Photography, Angela Elliott Design | Photography, Natalie Lynn Photography, Capturesque Photography, Trevor Howell 323 Photography and 180 Photography

Staff Writers:
Kat Painter, Leha Long, Laura Mak Quist, Sherry Goggin, Jodi Tiarht, Natalie Lynn Lichtenbert, Nicole Moneer Guerrero, Dr. Krista Bragg and Kenneth Bragg

Contributing Writers:
April Branton, Alyssian Vissat, Chandra Whitaker Cobb, Dennis Mason, Dr. Sara Solomon, Jenna Lobos, Joel Mosely, Linda Okwor, Keri Lynn Ford, Monique Kabel, Kimberly Miller, Miranda Hoffmann, Patty Wilson, Shelly Cannon and Vince Del Monte

Models:
Jodi Tiarht, Jennifer Wade, Laura Mak, Kat Painter, Keri Ford, Mary Boyer and Chandra Whitaker Cobb

Wardrobe:
Laura Mak, www.makattackfitness.com
Sherry Goggin, www.fitgirlwear.com

MISSION STATEMENT:

FitnessX Magazine strives to inspire all women by making a difference in empowering and encouraging them to live a healthier lifestyle. We take pride in sharing inspiring articles and facts on health, fitness and wellness.

Our readers vary in age, body composition, ethnic background, economic status, and professional background, but have the common goal of improving themselves through health, fitness, and wellness. FitnessX Magazine readers are health-conscious, discovering or already adopting healthy lifestyle practices, and interested in bettering themselves.

FitnessX Magazine features athletes in all sports, professionals who work in the health/fitness/wellness industry, everyday women who have made remarkable strides in motivating others to live a healthier lifestyle, and includes articles on the latest and most popular topics of interest.

At FitnessX Magazine, our tag line says it all—
"Inspiring YOU to Live Well…*NATURALLY!*"
Kat Painter & BillyBow

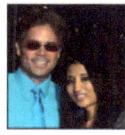

PUBLISHERS:
Kat Painter and BillyBow

The
Power
Behind
Mental
Strength

EDITOR-IN-CHIEF

PHOTO BY: BillyBow Photography

It's one of those week's with long hours at work, tons of errands, etc...and before you know it, you have no time to work out at the gym. On top of all that, you gave in to the temptation of eating off your meal plan. Not just once, but more times than you care to admit. I'm sure you've experienced this, at some point, with your workouts and nutrition. Whether you are new or a veteran in living the healthy lifestyle, it all boils down to how you face adversity. Will you buckle down under pressure or take the bull by its horns?

Ultimately, this is when your mental strength is truly tested. You've heard this inspiring quote, "When the going gets tough, the tough get going", but what really helps us get through the tough part in any situation is our own determination.

Mental strength is a decision. A mindset. Ultimately, you must choose to either accept ownership of your internal state and how you perform, or without this inner resolve. Make the choice and learn how to build on your mental strength with your own health and fitness goals! Sometimes, you have to make mistakes before you realize what works best for you.

Ask yourself -- "Do I feed my mind with positive fuel every day and push myself beyond my comfort zones?" If not, you'll want to start building your mental strength by developing a stronger focus and transforming limiting or negative thoughts. Your thoughts form a basis for your life and determine the way you see yourself in the grand scheme of things. Make it your mission to strengthen your mind, change unproductive habits and improve limiting perceptions.

Based on my own personal experience, my feelings have always had a strong affect on my performance. If I was in a bad mood, I knew the outcome would not be the best. Whether you are aware of them or not, how you feel affects how you perform. The mind is more powerful than the physical body. The power of the mind plays a significant role on your feelings about a particular event or situation. The message here is quite simple - learn how to change your interpretations and you learn how to manage your emotions. When you can manage your emotions you can perform at your very best.

With that said, get your mind 'in the zone' with your healthy practices. Train strong, eat well, and get plenty of rest. With a strong mind, anything is possible. Remember -- No one is perfect, so don't expect perfection. Instead, strive to be your best every single day! Don't ever give up on your goals! Ask for help when you need it. Hard work always pays off and gives you a wonderful sense of accomplishment. You are worth the effort!

At FitnessX Magazine, our mission is to publish the most inspiring articles from top fitness professionals and enthusiasts. We select our writers knowing that they possess the integrity and dedication to health, fitness, and wellness. Their desire is to inspire you (our reader) to live the best way you can and continue with your journey for self improvement. Remember that we are here to help you be healthy and happy! Feel free to e-mail your comments to editor-in-chief@fitnessX.com anytime! I am looking forward to hearing from you!

Inspiring YOU to Live Well...Naturally,

Kat Painter

Submissions:
For all Submissions, email submission@fitnessX.com and for rules & guidelines, go to fitnessX.com. Click on Guidelines for Submission at www.fitnessx.com/writers/.

Bikram Yoga & Competitive Fitness

WRITTEN BY: Shelly Cannon

These are two of my great loves. Apparently, I like pain and pushing myself beyond my limits. I have been practicing Bikram yoga about 7 years, and competing a little over a year.

Here are the top 10 benefits I receive by combining yoga with my weight training:

1) Muscle soreness relief - Nothing relieves my muscle soreness the day after a big lifting session than 90 minutes of stretching in a heated room. I can go back the next day to train hard and strong – much more than I would have without a yoga session.

2) Stress relief - We all know about cortisol and belly fat and the benefits of minimizing it. When I walk out of a class, I feel amazing - like nothing can touch me. This effect lasts about 3 days for me. When I start to get anxiety, I know it's been too long since I've been to a class.

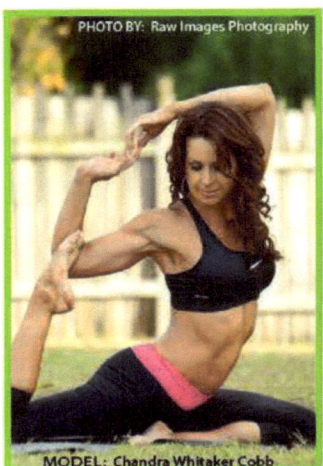

PHOTO BY: Raw Images Photography

MODEL: Chandra Whitaker Cobb

3) Increased Body Awareness/Motivation - Nothing motivates me more for my weight training than spending 90 minutes looking at my body from every angle wearing next to nothing. I get a good look at the areas that need more attention and I get confirmation of the results of all the hard work I've put in so far.

4) Cardio/calorie burning - I have done research on many sites and plan to test it with a waterproof heart rate monitor, but the online calculators agree that for my 115-pound body, I burn about 760 calories in a Bikram session. This sounds like a lot, but if you know how high the heart rate gets with the combined heat and difficult postures, you might think this is an understatement. I will update once I've tested it definitively.

5) Detox/water weight reduction/ph levels - I don't think anyone understands how much sweat we're talking about in one of these classes unless they've experienced it themselves. Any bloat from sodium intake is instantly gone. My pH levels always go more alkali by a large amount after a session. I drink at least a gallon of water during and immediately after class and feel amazing.

6) Mood boost - When I am heavily restricting my food intake, I can get irritable from time to time (hehe). A yoga class instantly makes me a more pleasant and happy person for a couple days after. I generally have a more positive attitude after a class, which is invaluable in the challenging world of competitive fitness.

7) Improved Sleep - We need good, deep sleep when weight training. I sleep my best and hardest after yoga. Period. I sometimes don't even move - wake up in exactly the same spot - covers unruffled.

8) Breath Control – Yoga teaches me how controlling my breath has different effects on my heart rate, mind, and body. I can use breathing to slow my heart rate, calm my nerves, energize my body, or relax. This is useful in all areas of competition, from training to stepping on stage.

9) Mind/Body Connection – Completing a yoga class puts me in better touch with my body. I have more of an awareness of where my body is, what it is capable of, and where it needs improvement. Bikram yoga teaches me that the mind is what really controls how strong I am or what I can do with my body. It trains me to use my mind to push my body further than I think I can go. This benefits me in all areas of my life, not just fitness.

Bikram yoga is not for everyone. It is hot, sweaty, time-consuming, expensive, and extremely challenging. But so is competitive fitness. Those willing to push themselves despite these hurdles are lucky enough to reap the benefits. In my opinion, combining the two exponentially increases the benefits of both. I hope to see more competitors use them together.

ABOUT THE WRITER: Shelly Cannon is *NPC National Bikini* competitor, fitness model and writer. She states, "I try to surround myself with positive people and am almost always smiling or laughing. Life is short and I'm making the most of every experience. I don't judge people and always remember that everyone's just trying to find some happiness in this world." You can contact Shelly at www.facebook.com/shellycannonmodel.
Photo by: Excipio Photograf

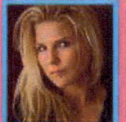

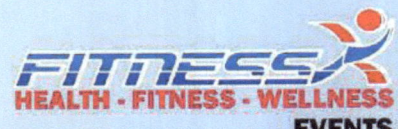

EVENTS

LA FITNESS EXPO 2012

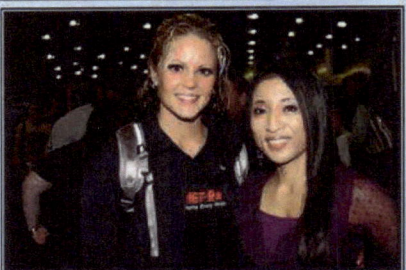

Nicole Wilkins and Kat Painter

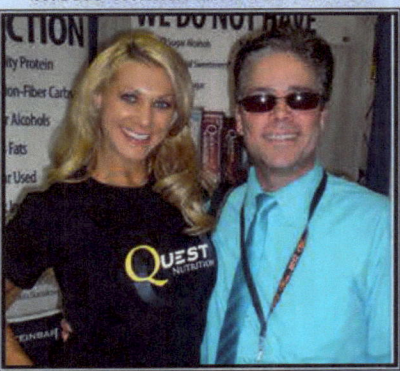

Jodi Tiahrt and BillyBow

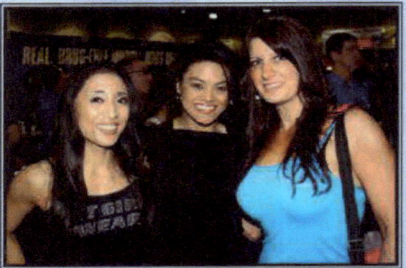

Sherlyn Roy, Leha Long & Kat Painter

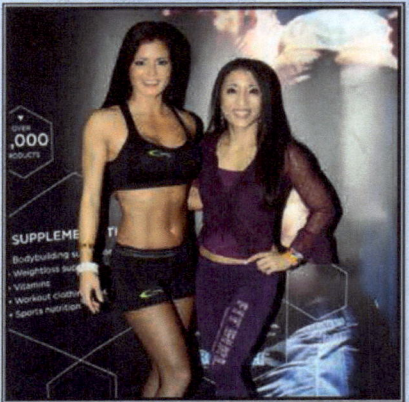

Stacey Naito and Kat Painter

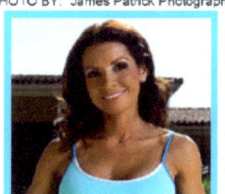

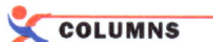

Don't Worry, Be *Happy!*

Written By Patty Wilson

In today's challenging world, it is up to us to create our moods. There is so much negativity that surrounds us daily and by changing how we handle situations and our thoughts we can change our lives.

My 10 simple steps to being happy:

1. Look for the positive things in your life right now. Live your life with positive optimism. Negative thoughts and worry zap your energy. Thinking of the good and positive things in your life generates feelings of warmth, affection, appreciation, hope, and security, and draw positive things to you. Also spend more time with positive people. Arrange to meet up with that friend who always seems to lift your spirits.

2. Show gratitude. Every day make a list of at least 5 things that you are grateful for in your life. Be happy with what you've got – not what you want. Focus on what is right in your life rather than what is wrong. Count your blessings and look at all the amazing things around you. Notice the little things we all take for granted.

3. Appreciate just what you have got going for you in your life right now. For example, stop obsessing about wanting a slimmer body and be grateful that you can walk. Begin today to tell all the people in your life how much you appreciate them being there for you.

4. Smile. Sounds simple but sometimes can be the hardest thing to do. Smile at everyone you see even strangers. The more you smile, the more people will smile back at you. Be prepared to be surprised at what comes back to you.

5. Make at least one friendly phone call each day, with no intention to get some business or anything else, just a friendly hello without any expectation.

6. Eat healthy and quality food. You need and deserve quality foods. Determine what food really works for you, and develop a personal way of eating that will support you. Do this because you are worth it.

7. Exercise regularly and make it fun. Take 45 minutes out of your day to work your muscles and strengthen your body, mind and spirit. Remind yourself of the benefits and adapt exercise habits as part of your daily routine of self care. Stop thinking of exercise as an option – start now and experiment until you find something you truly enjoy.

8. Get sufficient sleep, which will keep you shining. Determine just how much sleep your body needs and make sure you get it. Avoid watching TV, reading, doing work in bed. Make your bedroom a peaceful place for you.

9. If you are down a bit, then let it all out. Laugh, cry, scream or anything else you get the urge to do, but do whatever it takes to let out the emotions you are feeling. You will feel so much better and lighter afterwards. We all need to vent at times.

10. Do something for someone else. Random acts of kindness are magical and giving of yourself is one of the best highs you can get.

In the words of Joel Osteen "You can be happy where you are."
Patty Wilson
www.pattywilsonfitness.com

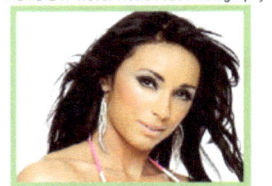

HAPPY Medium

WRITTEN BY Monique Kabel

— n

a course or state that avoids extremes

Finding your happy medium has often been said to be the pinnacle of successful living. Often enough we find ourselves pedal to the metal in either one or all areas of our lives. Our workloads become un-bearable; they spill over into our home life. The frustration of a chaotic home is projected onto our co-workers. We don't know where to draw the line and finish one thing, before starting another, leaving us going a mile a minute as walking talking time bombs.

For as long as I can remember, I have always gone at a turbo speed. Trying to accomplish as much into a 24-hour time frame, as humanly possible. I rushed to do everything, I rushed so much, and eventually I found myself stuck in high gear. It was almost like my life was in a state of panic. If I did not finish my daily duties by the appropriate time, the sky would fall…. Let me tell you, the sky isn't falling, and while it does take a certain amount of good time management, daily tasks can be done without speeding through them.

I found myself not enjoying anything anymore, and I decided I needed to find my happy medium and start living my life, not racing through it. Funny thing is, when I decided to slow down, I started to appreciate things so much more. I saw the beauty in the sunrise sitting in early morning traffic, I actually tasted my coffee for once, AND my stubbed toes and kitchen injuries were lessened greatly.

I'm not saying everyone needs to go home and meditate for an hour after work, although that would be ideal to have that sort of free time, but if we can slow down, at least for a moment or two, we would be able to see the beauty that surrounds us.

It's Here!

NOW you can READ *FitnessX Magazine* on your iPad, iPhone, Android & Kindle Fire!

Download the Kindle App from your phone app store for free! Then, you can read the FitnessX Magazine on iPad, iPhone, Android and Kindle Fire!

Go to Amazon.com -- in the search box type FitnessX Magazine!

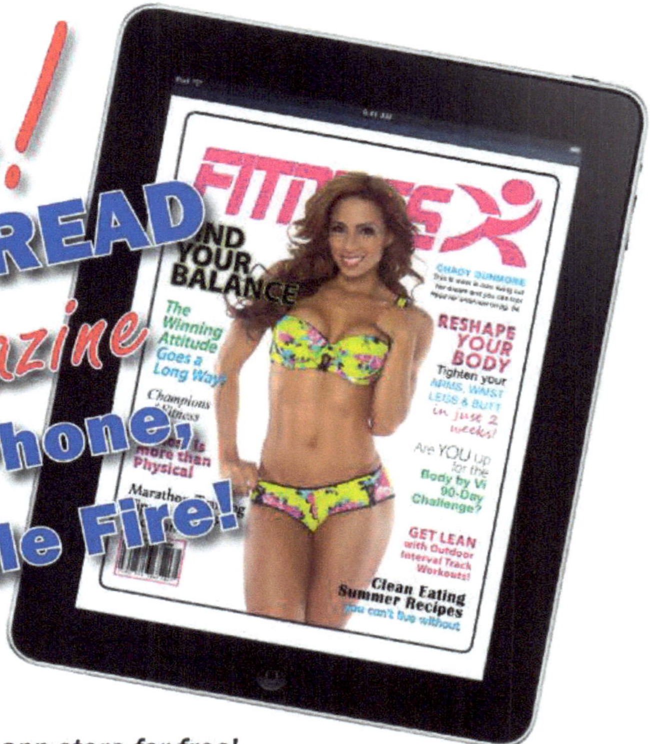

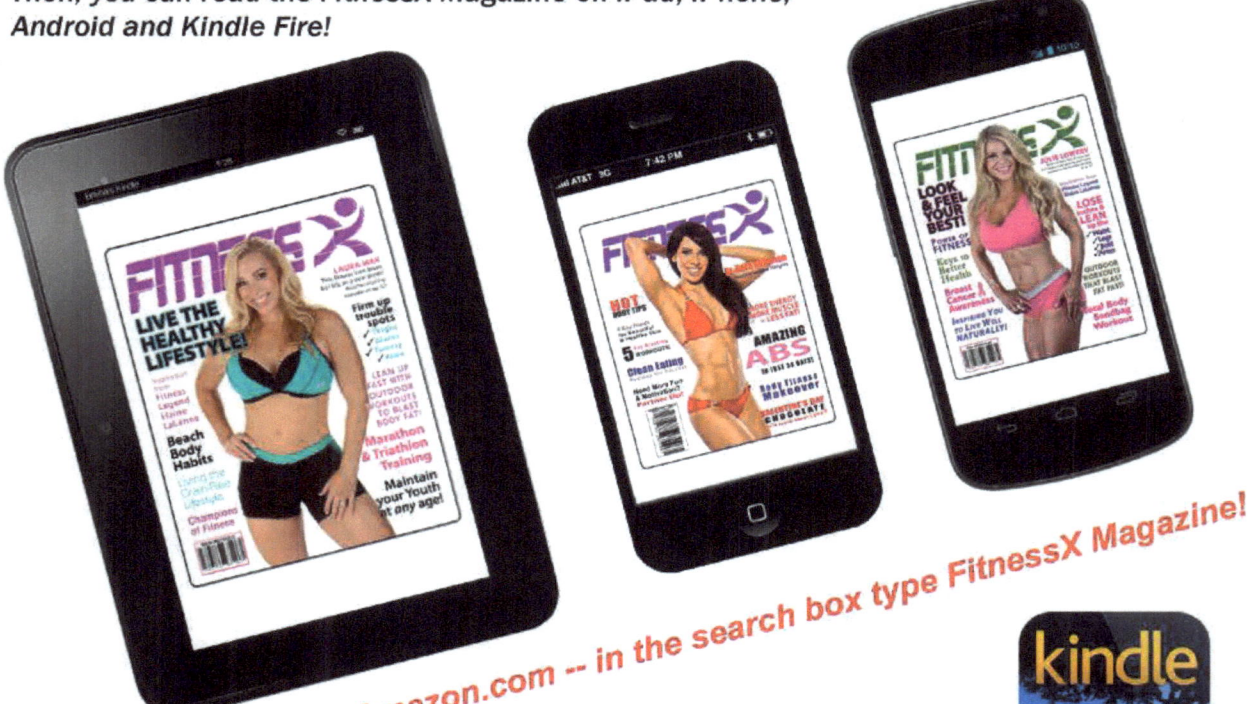

Just got off work. Looking forward to an intense back workout to take my mind off everything. I arrive at the gym, change into my gear. Madonna blasting in my ears. I strap my Zebra G-Loves on. It's go time!

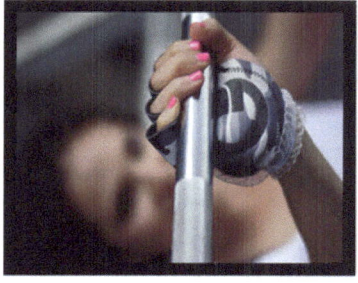

I start with 5 pull-ups. Beat my record. No slip grip in full effect! I move from the seated row to dumbbells. I'm in the zone – passionate and focused on goals.

My hands are feeling protected! I get a firm grip on the rear delt machine. My back is feeling tight. Just the way I love it!

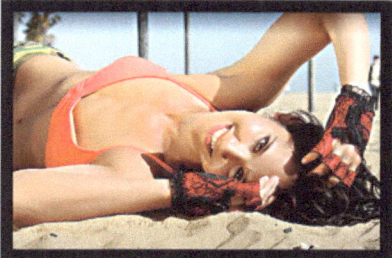

A woman strikes up conversation as I'm taking off my gloves. She's says I look "glamorous" in them. "And they can handle my hardcore workout!"

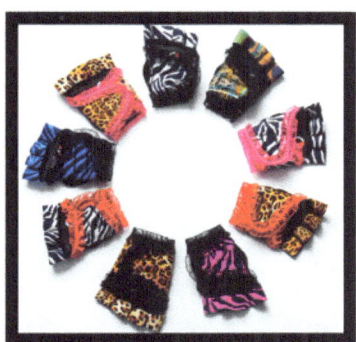

I reply, "My hands are smooth and soft. There is no pain in the hand." G-Loves are the ultimate workout glove for the fashionista athlete.

Tomorrow, I think I'll wear my Leopard G-Loves for chest day!

www.G-LOVES.com

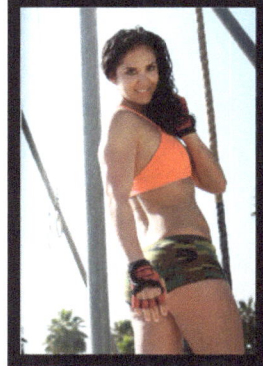

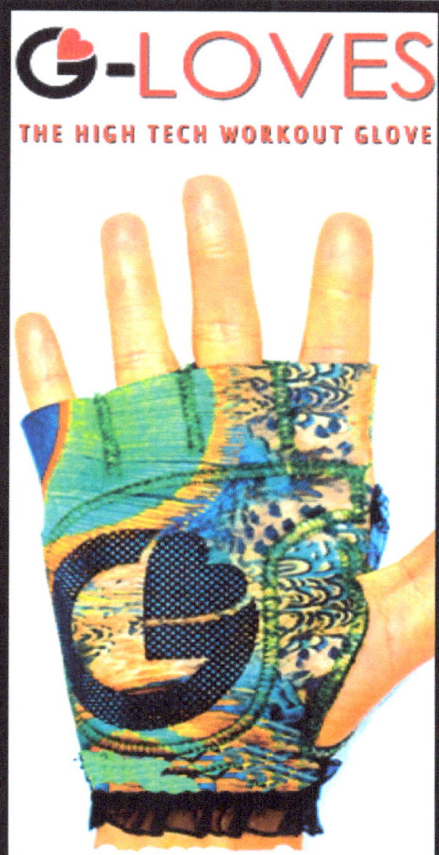

Get Your Mind *Right!*

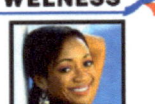

WRITTEN BY: Linda Okwor

I clearly remember sitting in the counselor's office while in school crying uncontrollably. I was not crying about a boy or my family, the reason seemed much more painful at that time. It was a scene that happened many times during those awkward years. I was crying because I hated my body. One of my peers just created a new nickname for my slim (lanky is more like it) frame. As a kid, you are picked on for many things but the taunts about my body often cut the deepest because I was reminded of it every time I looked in the mirror. I hid behind baggy clothes and often shied away from opportunities. We all have our own personal struggles. Regardless of what the source is, the pain is real.

My life changed when I discovered that I could reshape my body, mind and life using sports, fitness, nutrition and support. As my body and confidence changed, so did my self-esteem and life. This is why I decided to pursue a career in fitness, nutrition and health. I am able to impact lives and it feels amazing. I know how it feels to not like who you see in the mirror. I was able to conquer my challenges and enjoy the wonderful life I was blessed with. My personal journey cultivated a desire to help others do the same.

My biggest transformation was not physical, but something that could not be touched or seen; It is an immense power that is often overlooked. My struggles with my body and self esteem, and eventual freedom from it gave me an appreciation for the power of the mind. The power of the mind and inner strength create our beliefs and our beliefs create our reality. The beliefs create thoughts, which in turn, evoke emotions. It is the emotions that create the need for action or the opposite as well as the fear in not taking action. The action or inaction produces the results...your reality. Whether you will succeed or fail is determined long before any action has been taken.

As a nutrition and fitness specialist, I am a witness to people's most intimate confessions, struggles and successes. The journey is joyful, painful, challenging and inspiring. Whether they are battling a health issue, desperately trying to lose weight or preparing for a fitness or figure show, the beginning starts the same way. The first step of my fitness or nutrition program is always getting the mind right. The following are steps that have helped many of my clients achieve and exceed their goals.

Get Your Mind Right:

1. Embrace the journey
A few years ago, I read the best-selling book "Seven Habits of Highly Effective People". One thing that always stuck with me is "Be Here Now". It is one of the many powerful principles used to empower readers of the book. Making the decision to live a healthier life is not always an easy one. Questions such as "why am I here", "I can't believe that I am putting myself through this", "how much longer", etc... will only sabotage your efforts. Your body only knows what your brain is telling it to do. If negative, self defeating thoughts are a mainstay in your head then your body will act accordingly. No matter how you came to the decision to change, be here now and embrace the journey. Hormones are chemicals that are created in one part of the body (the brain) and transports messages to another part (the body). Your brain often sends messages to parts of the body using hormones as messengers. Use the messages to work in your favor by recruiting the appropriate mental thoughts.

2. Leave the baggage behind
When entering a new relationship, you wouldn't bring the pain, doubt, fear and augments of the past relationship? It is for the same reason that you wouldn't bring baggage from failed programs and attempts to your new program. We are no strangers to fads, get thin quick ads and miracle pills. By the time a client gets so fed up that they seek the help of a health professional, they have at least one failed attempt. If you focus on what is wrong or did not go your way, you will probably fail again. As a young hurdler when I was in school, I discovered that my fears often became a reality on the track. If I was pre-occupied with falling or hitting a hurdle, that was exactly what happened. I learned to visualize the best possible outcome. Those positive thoughts helped me cross the finish line more victorious than the "please don't let me _____" thoughts. Fill your mind with the best possible outcome, put fears aside and toss that failed attempt in the trash and you will see your goals accomplished.

3. Set goals
Some people feel unsure of what they are doing, some are frustrated by their lack luster accomplishments and others quit without realizing their full potential. One reason for the above outcomes is the failure to set formal goals.

Would you embark on a major trip without knowing where you are going? I wouldn't. Some may enjoy the adventure but an aimless trip can cause great frustration and loss of money and time.

Setting goals gives you long-term vision, short-term motivation and clear steps. It focuses your acquisition of knowledge, and helps you to organize your time and your resources so that you can make the very most of your life. Goal setting is used by highly successful people in all fields.

By setting SMARTER goals, you can measure and take pride in the achievement of those goals, and experience small successes along the way to get push you through the bigger journey.

When setting your goals, start with the SMARTER method. Goals must be:
- **SPECIFIC**
- **MEASURABLE**
- **ATTAINABLE**
- **REALISTIC**
- **TIMED** (date you will accomplish the listed goals) I added two extra acronyms that are valuable and worth implementing, E and R.
- **EXPECT** challenges because life will sometimes through you a curve ball. Just remember that failure is not falling but staying down. If you stumble, pick yourself up and keep moving.
- **REWARD** yourself for your accomplishments.

When you do something great at work, one can expect a raise, promotion, recognition or pat on the back. You can also pat yourself on the back for personal milestones. Decide on a reward system for yourself and which milestones to recognize. When you achieve those milestones, kindly reward yourself. Implementing these goal setting steps will help you set clear and achievable goals.

4. Identify challenges
Challenges can be overcome when identified and tackled properly. Take a piece of paper, turn it so the paper is wider than it is long, draw two long lines to create three even columns. At the top of the first column, write "Challenges". The second column should be labeled "Source". The third column should be labeled "solutions". List all your challenges, and then take one challenge at a time. In the second column, list the source of the challenges: long days at work or buying unhealthy snacks for the kids. In the last section, begin to list every possible solution that pops in your head regardless of judgment. Possible solutions can include taking lunch time walks, salsa dancing with your partner to combine a night out and exercise, playing an active video game with the kids, working out in the morning before work, buying healthy alternatives to unhealthy snacks or stashing sinful foods out of sight so you are not tempted to eat them.

After this brainstorm, pick 3 viable solutions for your challenges. Begin applying these solutions. You will find that the exercise of taking these items out of your head and onto something you can see will give you a sense of liberation. Listing solutions to your obstacles will empower you and provide solutions that you can apply to help you move forward. Try your solutions out and if one does not work, move on the next.

(Continued on page 21)

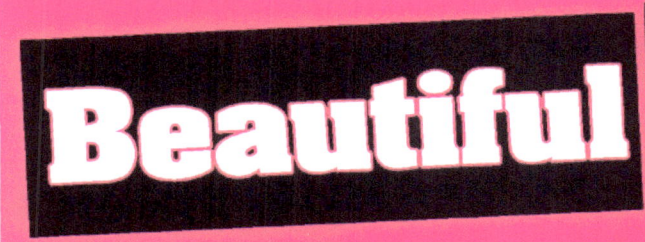 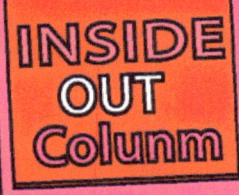 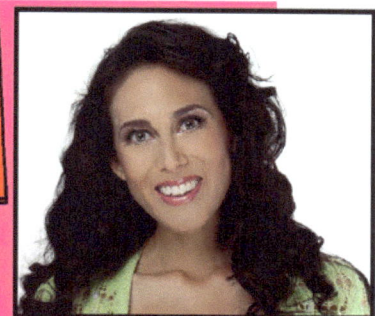

Beautiful INSIDE OUT Colunm

By Jenna Lobos

THE NAKED TRUTH

Q

Dear Jenna,

I am a business women, who entertains clients often, which includes going out to dinner and lunches. I would like to cleanse my body and partake in a detox, is there a way of doing so, without going on an extreme juice or water fast, and still go out with my clients?

+ A

Dear Marilyn,

This is a great question; although there can be some benefits to juice fasting, this does not always fit into a busy lifestyle. A simple and effective way to detox is through foods high in nutrients, this allows the body to detoxify itself naturally, the way it was meant to. Start with incorporating natural diuretics, such as kale, tomatoes, cucumbers, carrots, cabbage, melon and asparagus - these are great for ridding the body of excess fluid.

Purchase organic produce, whenever possible. Avoid the culprits; gluten, soy, dairy, and sugar, which can cause allergies. For your lunches, stick to lots of fresh vegetables and salads, which will keep your energy levels high. For dinner, you can add a non-toxic meal, such as roasted fish with kale or brussle sprouts. (Option: switch lunch and dinner) Tip: start your morning with one cup of aloe vera juice, 1 squeezed lemon, and 1 tsp. of *Udo'S 3-6-9 Oil Blend*. This will alkaline your body for the day, is great for digestion, and the healthy fats in the oil will slow down the absorption of any sugars that enter your blood stream. Make sure you keep hydrated with water, herbal teas, or aloe vera with lemon. Get plenty of rest, since your body has a difficult time getting rid of toxins when it is sleep deprived. I recommend keeping to this plan for 30 days, and then for 10 days each spring, summer and fall. This will keep your body clean and free of unwanted toxins. To your beauty!

Asparagus: It includes asparagines chemical. This chemical removes waste from the body by breaking up the oxalic acid. It also affects the cells and break down fat.

Cucumber: It is better source of sulphur and silicon. These minerals work to kindle the kidneys to wash out uric and unnecessary acid. It helps to stimulate the removal of fat, and loosens the fat from the cells.

Carrots: These have an abundant source of carotene which velocity the metabolic rate of the body and remove fat dumps and dissipate.

Kale: This is another salad food which contains water. It also holds iron and magnesium. It helps to wash out fatty cells.

Tomatoes: These have high water content and rich in Vitamin C that helps the metabolism and discharge of water from the kidney to swill down waste.

Cabbage: This is source of sulphur and iodine. It helps to purify the mucous membrane of the stomach and intestines. In addition, it assists breakage of fatty deposits particularly around the abdominal region.

Melon: Watermelon and muskmelon contains high levels of water, potassium and sodium that aid remove toxins and stimulates urine production.

What are some ingredients you should avoid placing on your skin? Do you have skin allergies or sensitive skin? Do you want to change your daily food habits, but need healthier alternatives? *Incorporate an organic and pure lifestyle from the inside out.* What we ingest into our bodies is just as important as to what products we place on our skin. The food we eat affect our moods, energy levels and overall well being. The products placed on our skin have a direct entry to our blood stream. Many items on the market today are loaded with toxins that cause hormonal imbalances, weight gain, fatigue, and much more. As a natural health practitioner, and following a 80% raw food diet, Jenna is an expert at what she calls "beauty foods". She will answer your questions on what foods to incorporate or what to substitute to provide you with ways to add living vibrant foods into your daily routine. A developer of her own organic, paraben-free skin care line, Jenna will answer questions on ingredients that should be avoided and how to become a mindful label reader. With a column that is dedicated to answering these crucial health and beauty questions, you will be educated and inspired to make simple, yet profound changes! To contact Jenna Lobos with your questions, email beautymarkgirl@gmail.com.

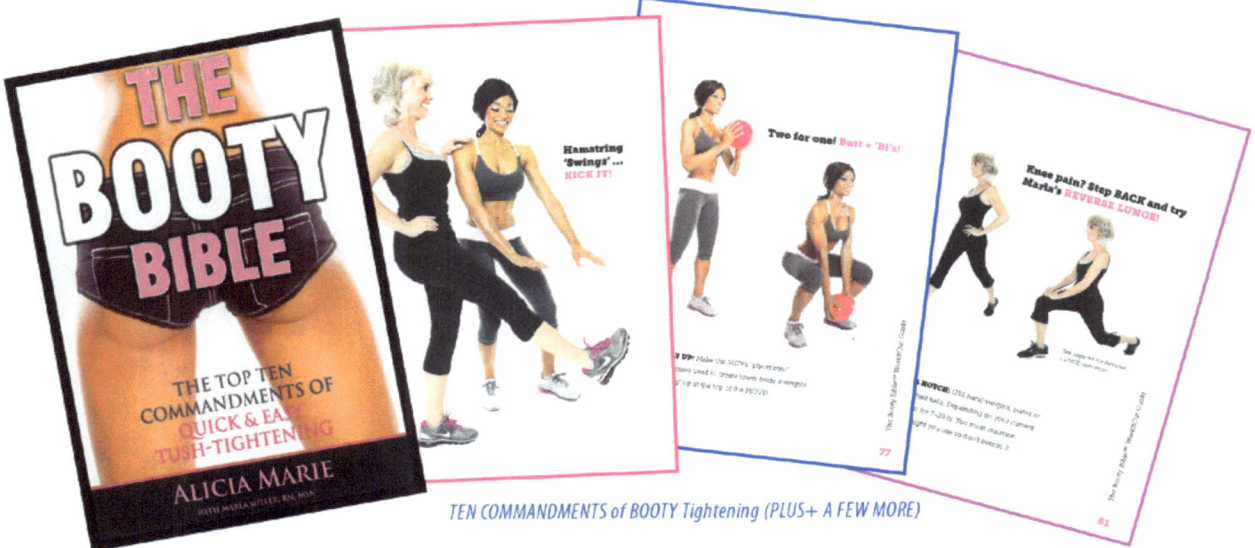

TEN COMMANDMENTS of BOOTY Tightening (PLUS+ A FEW MORE)

ALICIA MARIE is an *INTERNATIONAL fitness supermodel* and veteran health lifestyle writer. Alicia Marie decided that she wanted to get into fitness at the age of eight after spotting a comic book shot of DC Comic's Wonder Woman kicking the pants off some bad guys - while decked out in star-studded little shorts.

Fast-forward a few short years (and even fashion runways) later and ALICIA is now a *published author (The Booty Bible)*, an internationally recognized television and multi-media personality, a magazine cover model, a fitness wear designer (Alicia Marie by Rogiani) and a celebrity health guru. Not only does she pen her own column, *ASK ALICIA*, for many magazines and websites like *Oxygen Magazine* and *Fitness Magazine*, to name a few, but Alicia also opened a couple fresh cans of whoop-booty on MTV: Music Television as a MADE fitness coach and as one of the featured health experts on "Kirstie Alley's My Big Life".

In addition to writing fitness books -- she is currently the Editor-in-Chief of www.fitPOP.com, a fun, informational fitness and pop culture web destination for women AND the star of her own health and nutrition video series, "Alicia Marie's CARDIO WORLD" (WATCH NOW on FitPOP.com or on the series' YouTube channel).

Alicia is a NASM elite fitness coach with a degree in Neuroscience from the University of Connecticut and she has completed Broadcast Journalism studies from Columbia University...and yes, that is her rear in the Jergen's body lotion advertisement!

GET LEAN TIPS & TUSHIE-FIRMING 'FABOOTYLOS' NUTRITION & DIET FACTS

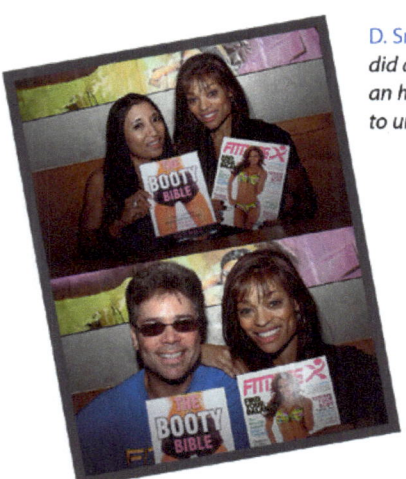

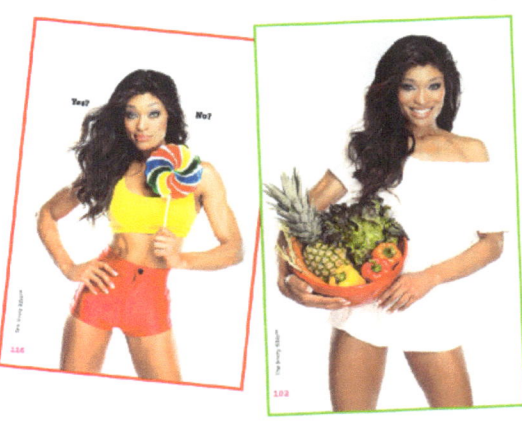

D. Smith writes: *"Fun to read! Alicia did a great job. Finished the book in an hour. Straight forward and easy to understand."*

Lauren writes: *"A fitness model that is more concerned with straight-shooting us mere mortals than filling a book with pictures of themselves and advertisements for the products they endorse. Alicia Marie is the best in the business, and she answers every question one could possibly have regarding getting in your booty shape."*

Go to Amazon.com to get "The Booty Bible"! $9.99

COMPETITOR'S CORNER!

WRITTEN BY: Leha Long   PHOTOGRAPHER: Angela Elliott Design | Photography   MAKEUP ARTIST: Pamela Pimpleton

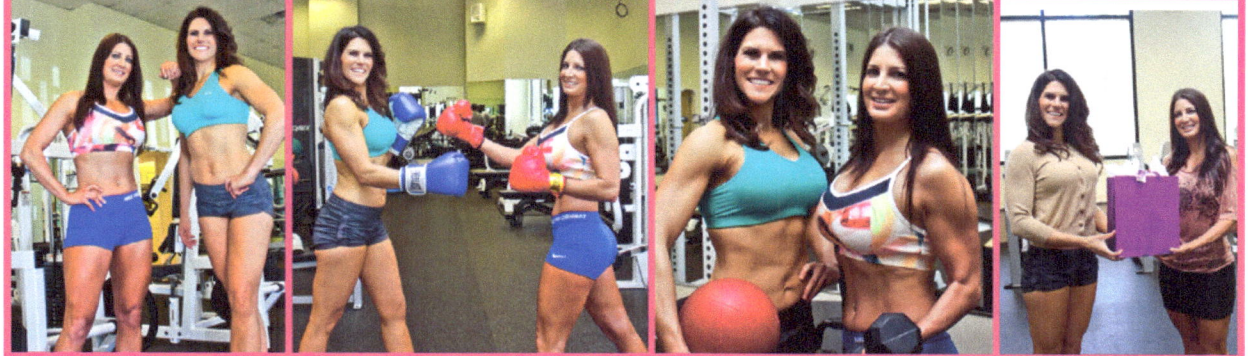

It's 2012, and time to prepare for another year of national competitions! My last competition was the *IFBB North Americans* in Ohio in September 2011. I happily placed 5th in my very first national show which motivated me for 2012! I plan on competing in a local show, in a couple of months, before my first national show to prep me for the real deal.

After my last show my coach put me on a less intense diet and workout. It is very important to give your body and muscles time to rest before shocking them again. During the holidays, I had to resist eating lots of sweets which is my weakness, however, I kept reminding myself not to overdo it, or I'll be spending more time at the gym working it off. I am now back on my competition diet with less carbs and my workout plan consists of more cardio. It's not easy, but I have my eye on the prize! My goal is to earn my pro card this year.

I have been very thankful for what 2011 brought me, and I can't wait to see what else will happen in 2012! I am very honored to have been on the FitnessX Magazine cover for January 2012 with America's top male fitness model, Greg Plitt. I've done a few radio interviews, appeared in some television shows and movies, and my clientele is building up.

Alot of people to ask me how I do all of this and how I got started, so I decided to write an article about it. They are usually shocked to hear that I do not have an agent and that I have done everything myself. My advice for those who want to become fitness models is to definitely get yourself in shape if you aren't already. Join a gym, hire a trainer, and eat healthy. Once you are in the best of shape, start competing to get your name out there. If competing isn't for you, then that's ok! You can still be a fitness model, even if you don't compete. Find reputable photographers who want to build their portfolios, and who will photograph you for free. Choose your best photos and submit them to various magazines and websites. You don't have to spend any money to get started. If you have a passion for this, then you will find ways and be creative to make it happen!

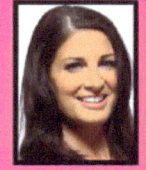

ABOUT THE WRITER: Leha Long resides in Atlanta, GA. She is a fitness model, national-level NPC Bikini competitor., writer, trainer, nutritionist and actress. Please check out her website at www.lehahealthandfitness.wordpress.com for more information.
Photo Credit: BillyBow Photography

I've been competing, writing, and modeling for almost two years now and would like to help someone else get started. Please meet the winner of the "Photoshoot with Leha" contest, Jennifer Wade! Jennifer is a wife, mother, competitor, and a teacher. She has been competing for two years now, and she says, "I hope through my story I can inspire other women to believe in the beauty of their dreams." I know with this attitude that Jennifer will go far. Best of luck to you Jennifer in the fitness industry! ✗

We would like to thanks Best Fitness By Pharr Gym in Atlanta, GA for providing the setting for our photo shoot!

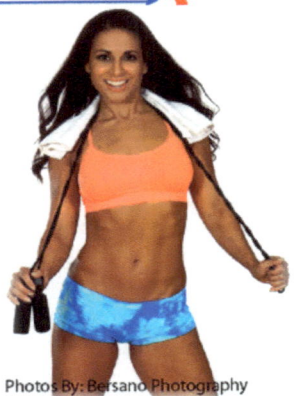

Nicole's *Glute Busting* Workout*!*

WRITTEN BY: Nicole Moneer Guerrero, NASM CPT for *Life Time Fitness*, C-ISSN IPPA, IFBB Pro

If I had a dime for every time I've heard the words, "I want my butt to look like yours", I'd be retired by now. There's a lot of debate on whether or not having a "badunkadunk" is genetic. In some cases this may be, others not. So there really isn't a definitive answer. What I do know is that in my own workouts, my client transformations and even seeing others progress, that genetics can be debunked with the right nutrition, weight training and cardio plans. You'll never know unless you get on a plan and most importantly are consistent for a minimum of at least 12 weeks. Consistency=Success.

Here are six of my favorite exercises that really target the glutes and leg muscles. If just starting out be sure to select a weight where you can maintain impeccable form. Once you master the form and can do 12 reps perfectly then I encourage you to gradually increase the weight. I always mix up my exercises, sets and reps each week or month. Remember if you do the same thing all the time you will get the same results. So don't be afraid to do 4, 5 and 6 sets instead of 2 or 3. If lifting heavier 8 reps may be all you can do without sacrificing your form and that's fine. Be sure to warm-up before we start building your bottom-half.

Photos By: Bersano Photography

1. Dumbbell Lunge from the floor up:

For this glutes and quad burning exercise exercise you'll need a mat and 2 dumbbells, initially you may only be able to do without weight.
- Place a dumbbell in each hand and assume a split stance (one leg in front of the other). Bend both knees to 90 degrees so you kneel on the mat on your back knee, this is your starting and ending position.
- Keep your shoulders stacked over your hips, drive through the front leg and heel especially as that really engages your glutes pushing yourself about half way up from the floor.
- Return to floor and repeat. Make sure to switch legs and perform on opposite leg.

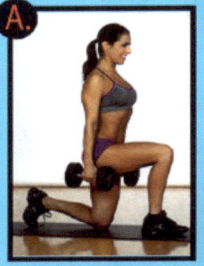
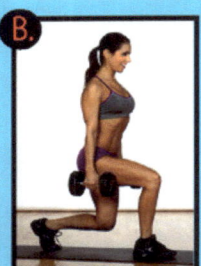

2. Single Leg Dumbbell Deadlift:

For this exercise you will need 2 dumbbells. You can also use a barbell, so mix it up!
- Start with feet in a split stance, arms straight with weight in front, this is your starting and ending position.
- Tip forward at the hip, keeping your back straight the entire time, make sure both toes are facing straight ahead (don't allow your back foot to turn out or in).
- Reach down as far as you can without rounding your back, then drive through your feet and heels to return to the top and repeat. Make sure to switch legs and perform on opposite leg.

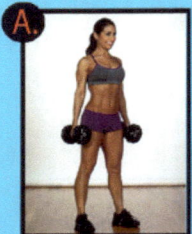
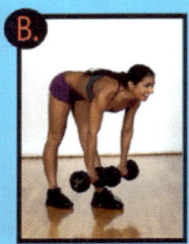

3. Single Leg Dumbbell Lateral Squat:

You will need 2 dumbbells or 2 weight plates for this killer glutes and adductor tightener.
- Start standing up straight with one weight in each hand feet hip width apart, this is your starting and ending position.
- Step out to the right with the right leg into a squat, all while keeping the left leg straight. The deeper you get into the squat the more you are really targeting the glutes. Aim to touch the floor with your weights if you can.
- Return to standing and repeat. Then switch to the left leg, stepping out to the left and keeping the right leg straight.

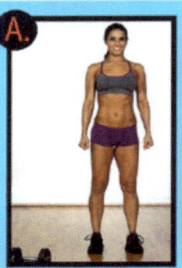
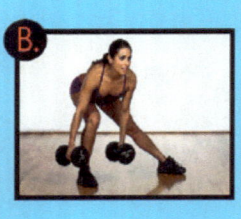

4. Single Dumbbell Calf Raise (from floor or step):

For this one you will need one dumbbell (don't be afraid to go heavy) and a wall to help maintain your balance. If you are more advanced, use a step.
- Hold dumbbell in right hand, balance on right leg with left hand placed on wall in front of you for balance.
- Standing up nice and tall, lift up onto the balls of your right foot and release back down in a controlled manner to the floor. Repeat on other leg.

To get an even bigger burn, graduate to standing on a step. Be sure to start with your heel dropped past the step

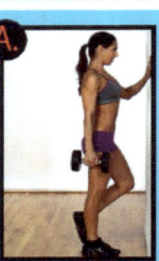
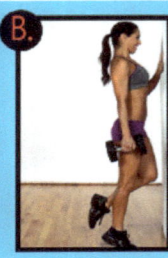

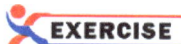

5. Single Leg Dumbbell Bridge on Bench:

This glute and core exercise will require a mat, a bench or box and dumbbells or a barbell. It can be done on the floor, but by adding in the bench or box you increase the ROM which makes it even more effective and tougher!

- Start in a supine position with feet on bench and your upper body on the floor, this is your starting and ending position.
- Place the dumbbells or barbell over your hips, extend one leg up so it's perpendicular to the ceiling.
- Drive the hips up to the ceiling, again driving through the foot especially the heel.
- Return to floor and repeat. Switch legs and repeat on other side.

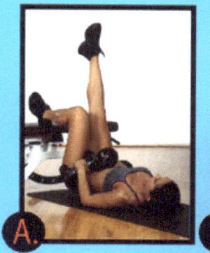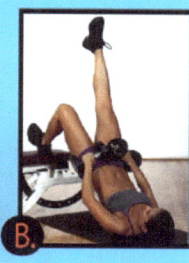

6. Stability/Bench Dumbbell Hip Extensions:

Grab a stability ball, bench and dumbbell for this butt blaster, for this one you don't need a lot of weight especially if this is your first time trying it.

- Place the ball on a bench, lay prone on top of it. Grab the bench with your hands to balance and place dumbbells between feet (you may need the help of a friend for this).

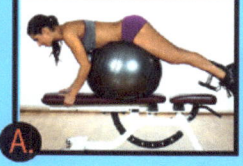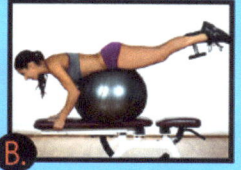

For more information about Nicole's background, client testimonials, online nutrition programs and more, please visit her at: http://www.nicolemoneer.com/ or "like" Nicole on her fb fan page http://www.facebook.com/nicolemoneerguerrero/.

ABOUT THE WRITER: With more than a decade of experience, Nicole Moneer Guerrero is an IFBB Pro Bikini Athlete, a Team Bodybuilding.com Athlete, a former Top 5 nationally and Top 10 internationally ranked fitness competitor and fitness model, as well as a skilled personal trainer and educator. As a NASM certified personal trainer, the 2009 Ms. Bikini Classic Universe Champion and VPX/Redline spokesmodel, her disciplined, results-oriented approach has garnered her industry accolades and it has inspired her clients to achieve their own personal fitness goals. Nicole holds a Bachelor of Science degree in Fashion Merchandising from Iowa State University. She resides in her native Chicago. For more information about Nicole's background, client testimonials and to refer to a full list of her competition rankings, please visit her online portfolio at www.nicolemoneer.com or on facebook at www.facebook.com/nicolemoneerguerrero. Photo Credit: Nicholson Studios

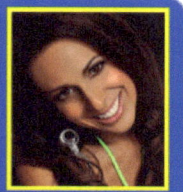

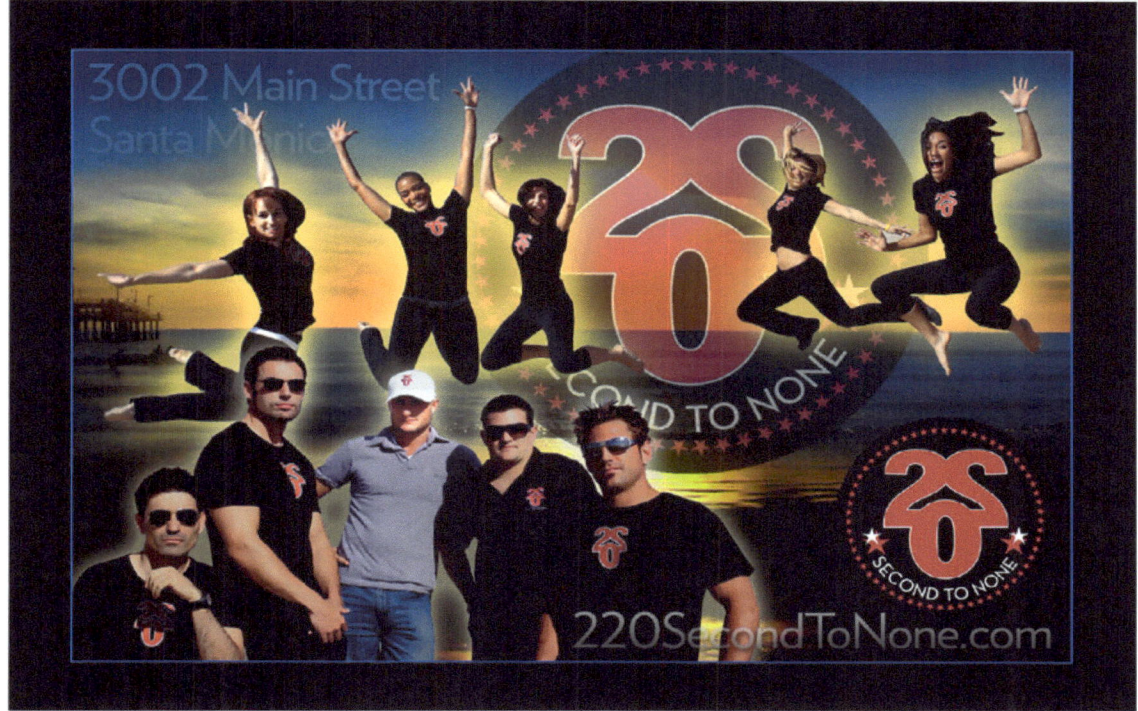

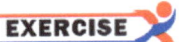
EXERCISE

Get
Tank Top Ready
with this
Arm Workout

Written By:
JODI TIAHRT,
CERTIFIED PERSONAL TRAINER

Photos By:
BILLYBOW PHOTOGRAPHY

Wardrobe By:
MAK ATTACK FITNESS WEAR
MakAttackFitness.com

Triceps & Biceps

With "tank top" season right around the corner, it's time to put the sweaters and winter coats away. With that in mind, comes sleeveless shirts and cute summer dresses. Give yourself an *instant makeover* by toning your arms. Because your arms and back carry less fat than the rest of your body; burning the fat off your arms can make you look "tank top" *ready* in no time! Follow this workout to build beautiful arms -- just in time for summer.

1. Skull Crushers

Lying face up on a bench with feet flat on the floor. Hold a barbell or EZ bar at arms length above your chest. Slowly lower the bar until it is above your frehead. Reverse the movement to raise the bar back to starting position. Repeat for a total of 15 reps.

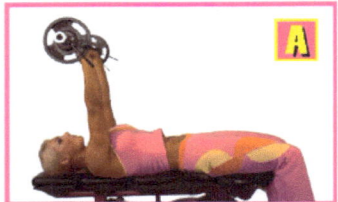
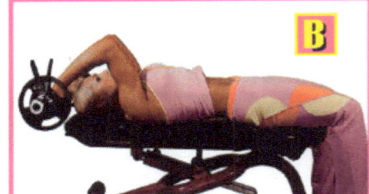

2. Barbell Curls

Starting with feet hip width apart, grasp a barbell or EZ bar with a shoulder width under hand grip. With elbows at side, raise bar until forearms are vertical. Lower until arms are fully extended. Repeat this for 10 reps. The next 5 reps, starting at the bottom, raise the bar only half way up so the bar is parallel to the floor. The next 5 reps, starting at the top, lower the bar only half way down so the bar is parallel to the floor. Now back to 5 full reps, starting at the bottom and raise the bar until forearms are vertical to the floor. This completes round one for a total of 30 reps with no rest. Repeat this 2 more times.

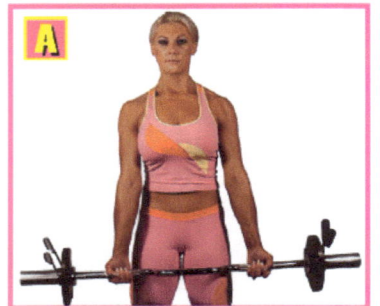
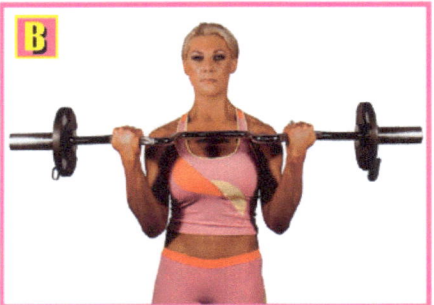
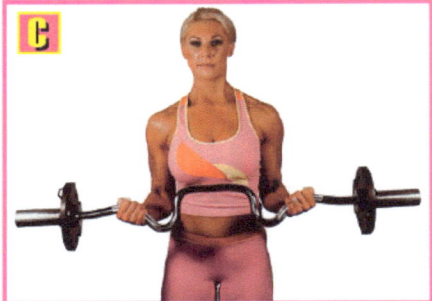

3. Dumbbell Hammer Curls

Starting with feet hip width apart, grasp 2 dumbbells at your sides with palms facing in and arms straight. With elbows to the sides, raise each dumbbell until forearm is vertical and thumb faces shoulder. Lower to original position and repeat for a total of 15 reps.

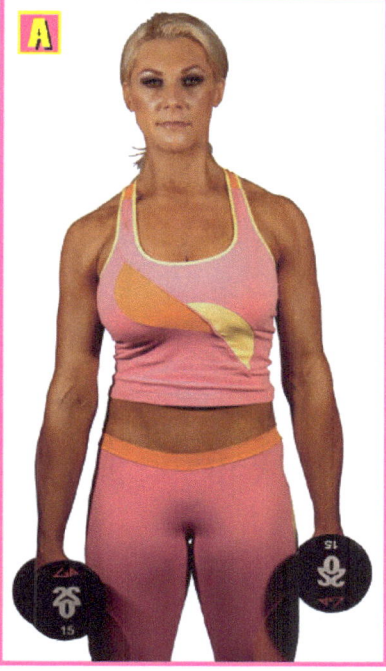
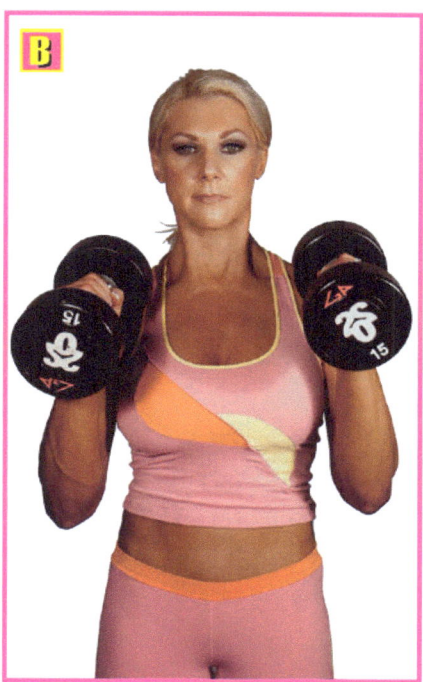

4. Bench Dips

Starting with hands shoulder width and feet straight out in front of you. Start with arms straight and lower your body by bending your arms at the elbows until upper arms are parallel with the floor. Raise back up to starting position and repeat for a total of 15 reps.

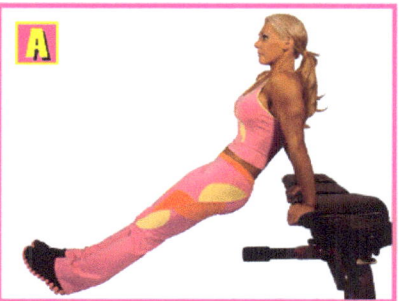
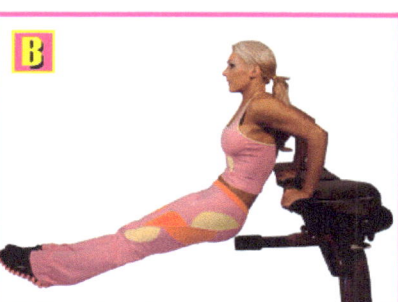

Skull Crushers, Dumbbell Hammer Curls and Bench Dips are 3 Giant Set exercises. These 3 exercises repeated in a row with no rest. Repeat these exercises for 3 sets. You will build beautiful biceps and triceps just in time for Spring and Summer! ✗

ABOUT THE WRITER: Jodi Tiahrt is a new *FitnessX Magazine* cover model/writer who excels as a fitness, figure, bikini and sports model champion. She has competed in over 42 competitions with 36 1st place titles. She is an international drug-free competitor having competed with the *ABA, INBA, Fitness America, Ms. Fitness, FAME* and *NPC* fitness organizations. As a life-long athlete, it was during high school and on through college, where she discovered her passion for health and fitness, which has become a lifestyle. Currently, Jodi is a certified *ISSA* Personal Trainer, Pilates & Fitness Pole Dance Instructor, Nutritionist, Motivational Speaker, Fitness/Sports Model and Actress. She also works as a spokes model and blogger for Quest protein bars, Haute Living Magazine and *FitnessX Magazine*. The multi-talented Tiahrt has over 10 years' experience in the field of personal training, nutrition, speaking, and is motivating and inspiring men and women of all ages through her unlimited accomplishments and ability. She defies the perception of women in the fitness industry as genuinely beautiful and feminine from the inside out.   Photos By: BillyBow Photography

How to Love the Skin that You Are In

Written By: Jodi Tiahrt

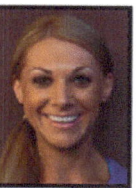

How many times have you flipped through the magazines and stared at the beautiful models only wishing that you could look like that? A lot of times we get wrapped up in trying to achieve an unattainable, airbrushed image of perfection. Let's face it, how many times have you seen a celebrity in real life and it doesn't even look the glammed up version in the magazines, television or even facebook. When we compare ourselves to these photo shopped images, we tend to get depressed. The only way to zap this negativity is to let go of unrealistic notions of what you should look like. Being fit and healthy means you not only look great on the outside, but you feel great about yourself on the inside. No one is perfect! Each and everyone of us has a unique set of talents that no one else has. We all have imperfections that make us unique. Accepting yourself and your body and loving yourself for the fabulous person that you are can lead to a more fulfilling life and a happier you. Put yourself first because you are worth it!

Try these tips to boost your self confidence and love the beautiful person that you are:

1. Focus on the positive.
Tell yourself everyday that you are a unique and fabulous person. Everyone has positive and negative traits about them. No one is perfect!

2. Replace negative thoughts with affirmations!
Buy yourself a affirmation book and read a couple pages every day. You will be surprised how great you feel after.

3. Accept your imperfections.
Stop dwelling on the things you can't change.

4. Talk to yourself in the mirror.
Say something good about yourself.

5. Don't worry about what other people think about you.
You will never make everyone happy. If you try to make everyone happy you will discover that others still are not happy and you have exhausted a lot of energy and you are not happy either.

6. Don't compare yourself to others.
Especially don't compare yourself to the images in the magazines.

7. Don't jeopardize your health to look a certain way. Starving yourself or doing a crash diet will only lead to bigger problems in the long run.

8. Pamper yourself.
Show yourself that you love and accept yourself. You are worth it!! ✗

HAPPINESS LIES WITHIN

WRITTEN BY: Dennis Mason,
Certified Personal Trainer & Fitness Coach

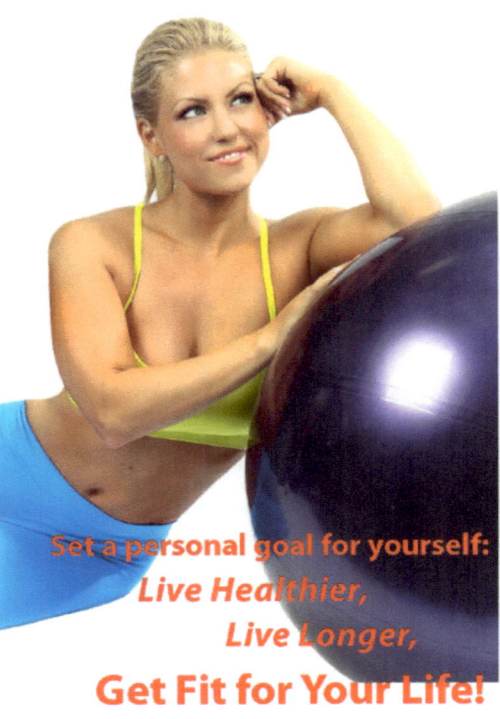

Set a personal goal for yourself:
Live Healthier,
Live Longer,
Get Fit for Your Life!

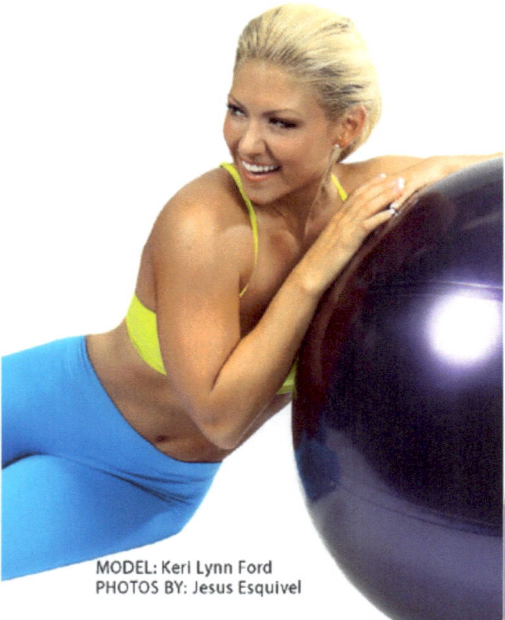

MODEL: Keri Lynn Ford
PHOTOS BY: Jesus Esquivel

Not long ago, I met one of my readers at a local party in Los Angeles. She told me that she was having difficulty dropping body fat for an upcoming photo shoot. She said she had been working out for about three years, but recently was not getting the results she wanted. So, she asked me what training routine and food supplements were the best for achieving a sexy, lean body. Her goals were to get firmer arms and a smaller waist. "If I can just reach these goals, then I will be happy," she said. Questions and statements like these are similar in nature to many that I receive. "If I had more shapely arms or firmer abs, I would be happy" is a common statement. Another is "If I just had the 'right' exercise routine, and the 'best' supplements, I could drop ten pounds off my waist." Unfortunately, this approach will seldom result in the level of success anyone wants with body shaping.

In our society today, we seem to have a set of 'desirable standards' of physical appearance for both women and men. These standards suggest that if you don't look like the people in the fashion magazines, or on television infomercials, or in printed advertisements, then you 'just don't measure up.' Generally speaking, these images are connected to some sort of commercial product, drug, exercise apparatus, or fitness center that will guarantee to give you the results you want, if you will just spend your hard earned money to purchase whatever it is that's being sold. The underlying idea here is that by achieving this desirable appearance 'You will look more attractive, make more friends and thereby, make you happier.'

Attempting to gain real friends or find true happiness is rarely the result of a product or a service. Very often the friendships that develop are superficial at best and the happiness of the moment soon wears thin. Then, it's back on the merry-go-round in an endless loop of searching for the 'best' anything to fulfill your desires. Deep down inside, you know that real friendship has nothing to do with the way you look. It's who you are on the inside that makes lasting friendships. Likewise, true happiness does not come from the outside, but rather from within. It comes through being in harmony and at peace with yourself. That doesn't mean that you can't have goals and aspirations in your life…it simply means using your intuitive sense to a greater degree when dealing with your personal level of fitness, health and happiness.

When I speak and write about a true 'fitness philosophy', I'm referring to a discipline that teaches us to achieve and maintain a healthy, fit and happy lifestyle. It is the combined awareness of our whole self (body, mind and spirit) that leads the way to achieving those results. Keeping the body toned and in shape is a lifelong lifestyle commitment. For example, all forms of performance expression, such as music, dance and singing, require that you know your medium, your 'tools' and the techniques needed to create the finished product. Working on your body is no different. In this case, your body is the medium. The types of exercise, foods and dietary supplements you choose are the tools. And, the methods of application are the techniques.

We are all blessed with the intellect that allows us to do what we need to do, use what we need to use and learn what we need to learn to turn our vision into reality. For example, if you choose to gain some muscle mass or lose some body fat, but are unsure or confused about how to accomplish those goals, our intellect tells us that we need to do some research on what to learn and how to proceed. On an even higher level, stay focused on the thought that you are part of the whole of 'all there is'. Be aware of what is going on around you. Allow the flow of energy to move through you and provide guidance in your life experience. Focus on your goals and maintain a positive mental attitude. Observe obstacles that restrict this flow and gently move them aside. In doing so, you will keep moving in a positive direction that leads you to the happy, healthy and fit lifestyle you seek.

Fitness is more than just a workout. It's a LIFESTYLE committed to staying active; eating healthy; reducing stress and having fun. Join me each week to be taken on a journey with me and my guests to explore new ideas; separate myth from fact and gain new information. That's *FITNESS & MORE* with me, Dennis Mason, every Saturday at 10:00 a.m. Pacific Time, only on Global Voice Broadcasting; www.gvbradio.com.

Set a personal goal for yourself: Live Healthier, Live Longer, Get Fit for Your Life.

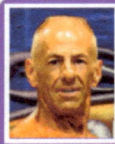

Dennis Mason is a certified personal trainer and fitness coach with over 30 years experience, an NPC bodybuilding competitor, charity cyclist, health and fitness motivational speaker, author, and talk radio show host. Contact him for information regarding his services.

On the Web at: www.DennisMasonFitness.com
www.FitnessAndMoreRadio.com
E-mail: dennis@dennismasonfitness.com
dennis@FitnessAndMoreRadio.com
On Facebook and Twitter: fitnessradio
Telephone: Los Angeles 323 207-5877
Palm Springs 760 219-5877

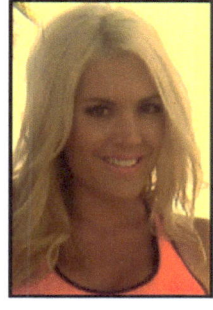

HEALTHY RESULTS
with
APPLE CIDER VINEGAR

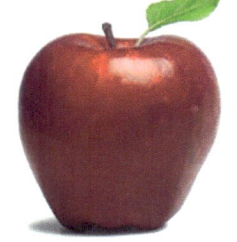

WRITTEN BY: April Branton

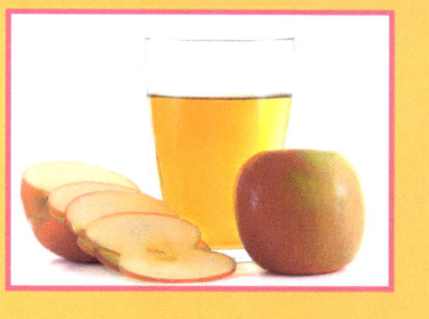

A serving of Apple Cider Vinegar a day keeps the fat away? Could losing a few unwanted pounds be as easy as ingesting a few measly teaspoons of a bitter vinegar? In case you were wondering, apple cider vinegar is a type of vinegar made by the fermentation of apple cider. During the fermentation process, sugar in the apple cider is broken down by bacteria and yeast into alcohol and then into vinegar. Like many types of vinegar, apple cider vinegar contains a substance called acetic acid proven to aid in weight loss. I know the bacteria and yeast is probably not sitting well in your stomach, but I guarantee the idea of shedding unwanted pounds can overcome any slight feeling of pessimism!

According to historical accounts, vinegar has been used for medicinal purposes for centuries. Hippocrates is said to have used vinegar as an antibiotic and Samurai warriors apparently used a vinegar tonic for power. During the U.S. Civil War, soldiers used vinegar as a treatment for various ailments including pneumonia and scurvy and was used to sterilize wounds during World War I. So apple cider vinegar has been around for ages and has apparently withstood the test of time.

Well let's begin with some scientific background on this wonderful vinegar, according to research, not only does apple cider vinegar help shed unwanted pounds but it also helps with all around health and wellness .For thousands of years, vinegar has been used for weight loss. Studies have shown that white vinegar as well as other types might help people feel full. A 2005 study of 12 people showed that those who ate a piece of bread along with small amounts of white vinegar felt fuller and more satisfied than those who just ate the bread. A report in the European Journal of Clinical Nutrition also showed that not only does vinegar help to control blood sugar and insulin levels following a carbohydrate-rich meal, but it helps to create a feeling of fullness . After ingesting just two tablespoons of vinegar followed by a carbohydrate-rich meal, the sense of fullness was more than doubled. These days apple cider vinegar advocates claim that all you need to do to lose weight is to take up to three teaspoons of apple cider vinegar before every meal. The vinegar has proven to help metabolize fat, and reduce your hunger and cravings. But does is actually help you lose weight? Remember the Acetic Acid I mentioned earlier? One small study (published in Bioscience, Biotechnology, and Biochemistry in 2009) found that overweight people who consumed acetic acid daily for 12 weeks experienced huge decreases in body weight. In tests on mice, another 2009 study (published in the Journal of Agricultural and Food Chemistry) found that acetic acid may help prevent the buildup of body fat and certain liver fats.

According to the Journal of American Diabetes Association an additional benefit is that a more acidic stomach may also increase the absorption of nutrients like calcium, magnesium, B vitamins and vitamin C. A 2006 study done on lab rats, showed evidence that vinegar could lower cholesterol and may be able to kill cancer cells or slow their growth. Scientists in Pakistan mixed apple cider vinegar with food given to diabetic and non-diabetic rats. Results showed lower LDL and higher HDL cholesterol in the non-diabetic rats. Similarly, the diabetic rats enjoyed significantly lower triglyceride levels and raised levels of HDL cholesterol.

So enough with the proof, you now know all about the health benefits of this wonderful fat-blasting , health promoting vinegar. But before you rush to the nearest store and stock up by the gallons, I want to let you know how to use apple cider vinegar to get the most out of it. There are a few ways to use it, by the teaspoon, while cooking or in pill form.

If you fancy the taste then taking by the teaspoon with not bother you. It is usually recommended to take two teaspoons a day (mixed in a cup of water or juice.) A tablet of 285 milligrams is another common dosage, you can find apple cider vinegar tablets online or in health food stores. And , if you wish to eat with meals a salad is the best way. I enjoy mixing a couple teaspoon's of Bragg's Apple Cider Vinegar with my favorite dressing to enjoy the ultimate salad! Now before you start chugging it right out the bottle (Caught you!) remember that apple cider vinegar is very acidic and can upset your stomach. It is strong and become harsh! Although it is said to be extremely beneficial with health and weight loss, always consult a physician before consuming. Remember to eat well and you can live well.

April Brandon's Recipes

APPLE CIDER VINEGAR

Ingredients:

Fat-Blasting Salad Dressing

- 3/4 cup olive oil
- 1/4 cup apple cider vinegar
- 2 tablespoons water
- 2 tablespoons honey
- 1 1/2 teaspoons salt
- 1/4 teaspoon pepper

Ingredients:

Apple Cider Vinegar BBQ Rub

- 1/2 teaspoon garlic powder
- 1 teaspoon sea salt
- 1 tablespoon Worcestershire sauce
- 2 cups apple cider vinegar,
- 4 ounces olive oil
- 2 tablespoons light soy sauce
- 2 teaspoons hot sauce

Directions:

Apple Vinegar Tea

1. Boil some water.

2. Put the vinegar and honey in a mug.

3. Pour the boiling water over it and dissolve the honey.

4. Drink and enjoy.

Keri Lynn Ford

A Firecracker on a Mission

Compiled and written by Tricia Anne Abernathy

PHOTO BY: John Lathrop

AGE: 27 YEARS OLD

BIRTHDAY: JULY 4, 1984

HOMETOWN: HACKETTSTOWN, NJ

HEIGHT: 5'0"

Every gal knows that our bags, whether it be a Micheal Kors hamilton, a Vera Bradley hipster or a Nike duffel bag, contain invaluable, and absolutely necessary items for our female well being. It is quite possible to get to know a girl solely by what is found inside these essential totes, don't you think?

Read on to see what things that we found in Keri Lynn Ford's gym bag.

The ipod

Recently Keri has been all about the FIT Radio app, specifically the DJ mixes of the "Top 40" genre to get in the workout mindset. Her latest iTunes purchase was "Glad You Came" by The Wanted. Artists ranging from Eminem and Rihanna to Linkin Park keep her going through an intense training or cardio session!

The crumpled up receipts

I was shocked to find that instead of some retail therapy evidence, Keri only had two receipts in her bag! A pet wash receipt from getting her 5-year-old Chow Chow/Australian Shepherd mix, Kaley, groomed and an airbrush tanning studio receipt she visited in preparation for her most recent photo shoot.

The grocery list

Keri usually loads up on clean eats from Sprouts Farmers Market including: chicken breasts, wild salmon, eggs (up to 5 dozen at a time!), red bell peppers, lean grass-fed beef, green beans, cucumber, Udo's oil, avocado, yams and oatmeal. Keri assured me that the one item you would NEVER find on her grocery list is cottage cheese.

Keri admits that every once in a while, soft serve ice cream with sprinkles and mini gummy bears will sneak its way into her diet...but not when she is gearing up for a show or photo shoot of course!

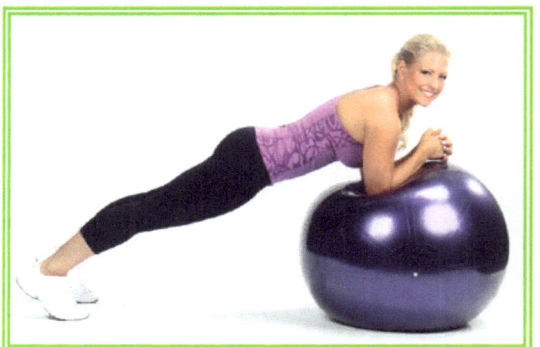

PHOTO BY: Jesus Esquivel

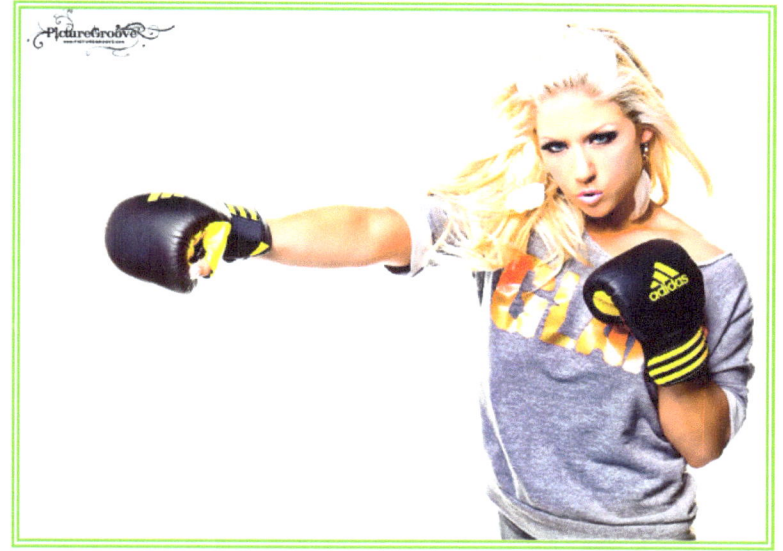

The wallet and ID card

Gift cards to one of Keri's favorite home décor shops, Pier 1 Imports, and her morning pick-me-up, Starbucks… even though she says she is more of Dunkin' Donuts girl. Her passport has the stamped memories of her study abroad program in London and a trip to Spain back in college. In the future, Keri hopes to add a stamp for Italy, where she hopes to meet her Italian cousins for the first time!

The workout journal

Treadmill arm walks, single arm tricep dips with a bicep curl and trampoline jumps. "I love training biceps and chest, but I am not really a fan of leg day!" Keri says.

The make-up for a fresh look all day

There are three items that Keri says are a must-have in her bag. First, she's a MAC eyeshadow fanatic, but the deep blue color "Contrast" is her favorite. Secondly, Victoria's Secret Beauty Rush Lip Gloss "Cupquake." Keri explains, "I love the color and it tastes like a sweet treat that isn't in my diet!" Lastly, Glam'eyes mascara by Rimmel to make sure to give her eyes that extra pop!

The supplements

Hands down her "go to" for protein powder is the organic plain egg white protein powder by Gifted Earth Originals because it is 100% pure protein! She also takes Glutamine, BCAAs and a multivitamin

The monthly calendar

First week of April: Check in with Coach Doug in Sacramento, CA

Mid-April: Tentative photo shoots with Sarah Lyons of Picture-Groove and Noel Daganta

Late-April: Representing Gifted Earth Originals and Eggology at Expo in Vegas

One last item that Keri explained is equally as important as her tote full of goodies, was her vision board of goals anddreams which she keeps next to pictures of her friend Rachael and her grandpa who both passed away. "It's to remind myself that life is short and I better be doing something I love every day," reveals Keri.

Keri Lynn Ford
GEO Sponsored Athlete, National-Level Fitness Competitor, Model + Trainer
www.kerilynnford.com
Follow me on twitter
Like me on facebook

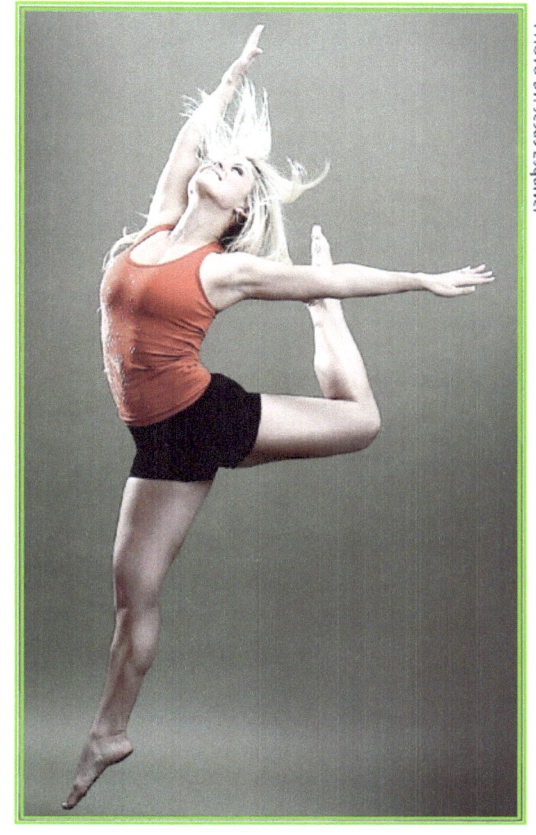

PHOTO BY: Jesus Esquivel

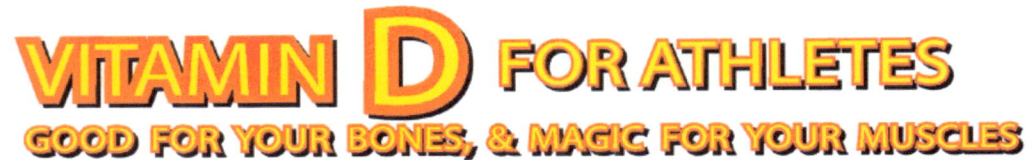

VITAMIN D FOR ATHLETES
GOOD FOR YOUR BONES, & MAGIC FOR YOUR MUSCLES

WRITTEN BY: Dr. Krista Bragg, DNP & Kenneth Bragg, RN

Well known as a regulating and absorption side-kick to Calcium, Vitamin D is a basic key ingredient to strong bones and teeth. An ace at multitasking, Vitamin D (technically a prohormone), plays a critical role in many aspects of our health and wellness. For example, Vitamin D deficiency has been associated with an array of health problems including: insulin resistance, glucose intolerance, arthritis, cardiovascular disease and even some cancers.

Vitamin D supplementation has been found to decrease influenza, the common cold, and even gastrointestinal infections by playing an important role in immune cell function.

Importantly, athletes who are devoted to building muscle size and strength may be interested in knowing the crucial role Vitamin D plays in muscular development. A variety of studies (man, animal, and cell) have all demonstrated that vitamin D impacts muscle function as well as strength. Vitamin D plays a vital role in muscle cell growth, cell stability, and muscle cell damage-control (J Steroid Biochem Mol Biol, 2011). In 2008, a comprehensive clinical research review concluded Vitamin D increases the size and number of Type II (fast twitch) muscle fibers and is directly associated with improved athletic performancen (Med Sci Sports Exerc). A large 2011 Australian meta-analysis confirmed that Vitamin D supplementation is consistently associated with increases muscle strength in vitamin D deficient subjects, although limited impact on those with normal levels (Osteoporosis International).

Randomized and cross-sectional studies have consistently demonstrated functional roles for Vitamin D in skeletal muscle. The relatively recent discovery of Vitamin D receptors within human skeletal muscle tissue further supports the role of Vitamin D in muscle function (Histochem, 2001).

Also, pertinent to competitors, researchers found a connection between increased visceral (belly fat) and low levels of vitamin D while another recent clinical study found lower levels of Vitamin D were linked to increased fat within muscles (Journal of Clinical Endocrinology & Metabolism, 2010).

Once considered a disorder of the elderly, the effects of Vitamin D deficiency are becoming more recognized in the younger population as well as athletes of all ages.

Signs of deficiency

Sports medicine researchers evaluated 98 dancers and athletes and found 73% were Vitamin D deficient (Clin J Sport Med 2010). Another study of collegiate athletes revealed, although Vitamin D deficiency was rare during the spring, summer, and fall, levels declined dramatically during the winter months (Med Sci Sports Exerc 2011). Researchers published in the Journal of Clinical Endocrinology and Metabolism found almost 60 percent of female study subjects were deficient in Vitamin D (2010). A 2011 Spanish study measured blood levels of Vitamin D in professional basketball players and found 57% with low levels (defined as deficient) after the winter months.

Signs of Vitamin D deficiency can include: heart rhythm problems, muscle weakness, bone pain, depression, and lowered immunity. Sometimes symptoms are vague. A simple blood test prescribed by your health care provider can reveal your 25-hydroxyvitamin D (Vitamin D) level.

Treatment

The healthiest treatment for any nutritional deficiency is generally via natural sources such as food. Supplementation should only be considered after a diet assessment and typically with the recommendation of your health care provider. The table below lists the Vitamin D contents of many common foods, as provided by the Department of Agriculture. Competitors may need to read this list closely as many dieting are not including fortified foods such as milk and cereal in their cutting phase, possibly allowing them to be more vulnerable to Vitamin D deficiency.

Sunlight

Well-known as the "sunshine vitamin", it makes sense most vitamin D synthesis is achieved through a reaction with sunlight on skin, specifically ultraviolet B radiation. In the 1950s, German coaches felt UV light acted as an ergogenic agent and were convinced athletes performed better (smartly so) and the use of sunblock with SPF 8+ interrupts the UV ray ability to stimulate Vitamin D synthesis.

Individuals with dark skin are particularly at risk because the presence of melatonin absorbs the UVB rays, which limits Vitamin D production. Those who live in areas of limited sunlight or have limited exposure may also require supplementation. Typically 15 minutes a day of unprotected skin exposure to sunlight is required to generate adequate amounts of Vitamin D.

Important to note, even populations in warm climates can be at risk for Vitamin D deficiency- one Brazilian study reported 60% of young people living in their sunny climate had vitamin D deficiency. Other studies also report that even in sunny climates, Vitamin D deficiency is frequent (J Clin Endocrinol Metab. 2010).

Latest Supplementation Guidelines

The average daily diet (non-bodybuilder/competitor diet) that includes fortified cereals and common foods is thought to only provide on average 250-300 IU daily. Athletes who are avoiding fortified breads and cereals may find their daily levels are even lower, particularly in winter months or low-sunlight climates. Evidence supporting the benefits of Vitamin D has been strong enough to prompt the Institute of Medicine to revamp its daily Vitamin D recommendations within the past couple of years.

In 2010 the Institute of Medicine released new dosage recommendations for Vitamin D supplementation. Based on an extensive review of research, the following doses are now recommended: Ages 1-70 years of age: 600 international units (IUs) per day. People older than age 71 are recommended 800 IUs. Vitamin D is typically found as Vitamin D3 or D2.

Interestingly, D3 is often considered a prohormone as by definition it is not technically a vitamin, but rather a catalyst for reaction that naturally occurs in our body.D3 (cholecalciferol) is often preferred and considered more clinically useful as most research has been based on D3 supplementation. D3 supplementation is considered less toxic, more potent, more effective, and more stable (lasts longer in the body) than D2. However, the preliminary agent for D3 synthesis is typically animal-based, which may not be desired by some vegetarians.

D2 (ergocalciferol) is more synthetic than D3 and felt to be less "natural" to some experts. However, as a fungal derivative, some vegans may prefer it to the animal product based-D3. Most prescription Vitamin D comes in the D2 form.

Dangers of Overdosing

Vitamin D is a fat-soluble vitamin, so there are valid concerns about toxicity from excessive doses. In addition, individuals with certain health conditions and genetic diseases may be harmed by Vitamin D supplementation, so checking with your health care provider is always recommended. Signs of Vitamin D overdose or toxicity include: headache, the taste of metal in your mouth, nausea, kidney stones and/or problems with your pancreas.

Summary

A blood test during your annual physical can determine if you are Vitamin D deficient. Until then, if you experience vague symptoms such as fatigue, depression, muscle aches, low energy (or the other symptoms mentioned earlier) and your diet does not include many Vitamin D fortified foods and/or you have limited exposure to sunlight, your levels may be low. Whether a dieting competitor or an off season athlete, your diet and lifestyle may not promote Vitamin D health; a simple blood test by your health care provider can let you know for sure!

Common Food Sources of Vitamin D	IUs Per Serving
Cod liver oil, 1 tablespoon	1,360
Salmon (sockeye), cooked, 3 ounces	447
Mackerel, cooked, 3 ounces	388
Tuna fish, canned in water, drained, 3 ounces	154
Orange juice fortified with vitamin D, 1 cup (amount of added vitamin D varies)	137
Milk, nonfat, reduced fat, and whole, vitamin D-fortified, 1 cup	115-124
Yogurt (amount varies)	80-90
Margarine, fortified, 1 tablespoon	60
Liver, beef, cooked, 3.5 ounces	49
Sardines, canned in oil, drained, 2 sardines	46
Egg, 1 large (vitamin D is found in yolk not much in whites)	41
Ready-to-eat cereal, fortified with 10% of the DV for vitamin D, 0.75–1 cup (amount varies according to amount of Vitamin D fortified)	40

How * IUs = International Units.

Note: The measurement IU = International Units and is an internationally used method of standardizing the contents of a dose of a particular vitamin. One IU of one vitamin is not the same content or dose as an IU of another kind of vitamin. For example, 1 IU of Vitamin D is not the same dose or milligram content as 1 IU of Vitamin B.

Source: U.S. Department of Agriculture, Agricultural Research Service. 2010. USDA National Nutrient Database for Standard Reference. Release 23.

(GET YOUR MIND RIGHT continued)

5. Affirm your thoughts

You know that the mind controls what the body does, but did you know that you can control what your mind tells your body? Through daily affirmations, you can positively effect the emotions and messages that your mind sends to the body.

Steps to writing and doing affirmations are:

1) Start with "I…"

2) Keep it in the present - "I am…"

3) Keep it positive - "I am blessed…"

4) Be yourself - "I am blessed to have kick a** work ethic."

5) Incorporate your goals - "I am happy to have lost 10lbs."

6) Don't focus on the how - "I am happy to have lost 10lbs."

7) Add current accomplishments,- "I am proud to have my college degree and a great family."

8) Make it fun - "I am a damn good cook."

9) Write multiple affirmations - "I am blessed, I am happy, I am proud…"

10) Say it many times every day. When you wake up, before bed, when you are feeling down, when you are feeling challenged, when you want ice cream, etc…

After repeated, consistent and continuous affirmations, your mind will have no choice but to believe that which you are telling it. Guess what? Your body will follow along as well!

Achieving your goals and living your best life begins and ends in your mind. The power of the mind and inner strength create our beliefs and our beliefs create our reality.

References:

1. Bescós García R, Rodríguez Guisado FA. Low levels of vitamin D in professional basketball players after wintertime: relationship with dietary intake of vitamin D and calcium. Nutr Hosp 2011; Oct; 26(5):945-51.

2. Bischoff H, Borchers M, Gudat F,Duermueller U, Theiler R, Stahelin H, Dick W. In situ detection of 1,25-dihydroxyvitamin D3 receptor inhuman skeletal muscle tissue. Histochem J 2001; 33: 19–24.

3. Chiu KC, Chu A, Go VL, Saad MF 2004 Hypovitaminosis D is associated with insulin resistance and β cell dysfunction. Am J Clin Nutr 2004; 79:820–825.

4. Constantini NW, Arieli R, Chodick G, Dubnov-Raz G. High prevalence of vitamin D insufficiency in athletes and dancers.Clin J Sport Med 2010; 20(5):368-71.

5. Dirks-Naylor AJ, Lennon-Edwards S. The effects of vitamin D on skeletal muscle function and cellular signaling.J Steroid Biochem Mol Biol. 2011; 125(3-5):159-68.

6. Gilsanz V, Kremer A, Mo AO, Wren TA, Kremer R. Vitamin D Status and its relation to muscle mass and muscle fat in young women. Journal of Clinical Endocrinology & Metabolism 2010; 95 (4): 1595-1601.

7. Gordon PL, Sakkas GK, Doyle JW, Shubert T, Johansen KL. The relationship between vitamin D and muscle size and strength in patients on hemodialysis. J Ren Nutr 2007; 17(6): 397–407.

8. Halliday TM, Peterson NJ, Thomas JJ, Kleppinger K, Hollis BW, Larson-Meyer DE. Vitamin D status relative to diet, lifestyle, injury, and illness in college athletes. Med Sci Sports Exerc 2011; 43(2):335-43.

9. Holick MF. Calcium plus vitamin D and the risk for colon cancer. N Engl J Med 2006; 354:2287-228.

10. Hyppönen E, Power C. Vitamin D status and glucose homeostasis in the 1958 British birth cohort: the role of obesity. Diabetes Care 2006; 29:2244–2246.

11. Matsuoka LY, Worsman J, Haddad JG, Kolm P, Hollis BW. Racial pigmentation and the cutaneous synthesis of vitamin D. Arch Dermatol 1990; 127:536–8.

ABOUT THE WRITER: Kenneth Bragg RN, BSN, BS is professional natural bodybuilder, personal trainer, bodybuilding and figure judge. He is published author of several fitness articles including *www.bodybuilding.com* and *Fitness and Physique Magazine*. Kenneth is the official host of *Natural Bodybuilding* cable television show (Adelphia 2000-2003).

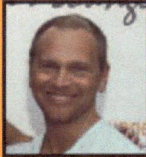
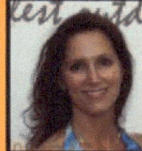

ABOUT THE WRITER: Dr. Krista Bragg, DNP is Certified Registered Nurse Anesthetist (CRNA) with a Doctorate in Nursing Practice, MS Nursing Administration, and MS Nurse Anesthesia. She is an Adjunct Faculty member from the University of Pittsburgh Graduate School of Nursing. Dr. Bragg is also a clinical author of health related articles, and nursing textbooks. She is an avid runner and noncompetitive bodybuilder. You can contact Krista at kristabragg@hotmail.com.

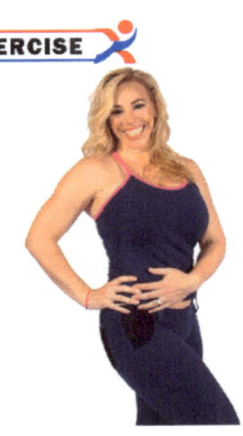

EXERCISE

Written By:
LAURA MAK QUIST, MS,
PREGNANCY FITNESS
SPECIALIST

Photo By:
BILLYBOW PHOTOGRAPHY

Wardrobe By:
MAK ATTACK FITNESS WEAR
MakAttackFitness.com

Welcome Back Abs - Getting into your Core Groove!

Abdominals,   Glutes   &   Lower Back

After the excitement of bringing your baby home settles into quiet contentment, (ha!) you may have noticed that you not only brought home a precious baby, but also a not so precious bulge in your belly. This is primarily because it takes your uterus a period of time to shrink down. Remember it took you nine, almost ten months to grow your baby and the belly just doesn't go away immediately after you deliver. But there are ways that you can certainly encourage your belly to strengthen and flatten. There are three important variables are that impact the shrinking of the uterus and the decreasing of the bulge. Of course, you need to remember to eat a healthy diet. If you are breast feeding, that will help you regain your shape at a faster rate as well. When you are able, a consistent exercise program should begin.

According to the American Congress of Obstetricians and Gynecologists (ACOG), it is typically safe to begin an exercise program three weeks after you deliver vaginally and six weeks if you deliver Cesarean (C-section). Listed below are five of my favorite belly exercises that reduce the size of the waist, strengthen the core, and give the flat appearance that we look for after the baby is born. Remember to check with your doctor before beginning any exercise program. These are the exercises I started to do about six weeks after my baby boy was born via C-section. My waist, belly, and hips have decreased several inches (just under three inches) from starting these exercises two weeks ago. This program has to be done regularly 2-4 times a week along with cardio, such as walking, and eating sensible healthy meals.

Here are five exercises that you can do to enlist the work of your abdominal muscles and gently get them back into the groove of not only functioning, but also giving you that trim waist line. It is important to gradually work into each of these movements and not to strain too much, especially if you have had a C-section.

1. Pelvic Tilt

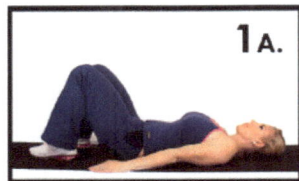

1A.

Advanced 1A.

This is the most important exercise of the five listed, because it engages the abs and core by gently moving the body without strain while strengthening. Lie flat on your back with your feet close to your hips and knees bent. Arms should be straight and out to the sides for support but not pressing into the ground. Begin with an inhale, and on the exhale, lift the hips up off the floor only about an inch or two. This is a very small and concentrated movement. The emphasis should be on pulling the abs in close towards the spine. On the next inhale lower the hips to the start position. Repeat this exercise for 20-50 repetitions. As you get stronger in this position you can do a variation movement and perform this at a faster pace, but not until you can do 50 reps comfortably. ADVANCED movement can lift the hips up higher into a "bridge" pose. To start the movement inhale, then on the exhale lift the hips up as high as you can pressing your pelvis towards the ceiling. Pause for a moment, then on the next inhale lower the hips to the start position. Repeat this movement for 20-30 repetitions.

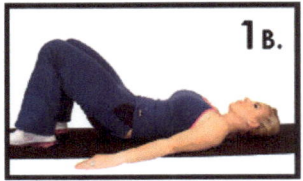

1B.

Advanced 1B.

3. Elevated Bicycle

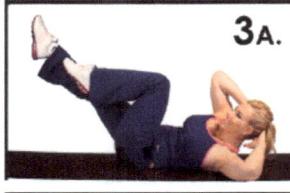

3A.

Advanced 3A.

Begin in the same position as the Core Heel Tap, but place your hands behind your head. Elevate your head off the ground. On the exhale, reach the right elbow over to the left knee and extend the right leg out to a 45-degree angle or higher (this may feel strenuous on the lower abs, so if it does, raise your leg even higher until the "strain" is not present). Repeat on the other side. Perform 20 reps on each side. ADVANCED movement will extend the leg to a lower position about 6 inches off the ground. Be conscious of how your abs feel in this position and just gradually change the angle to a slightly lower position. Try to challenge yourself by lowering your leg a few inches on a weekly or every two week period.

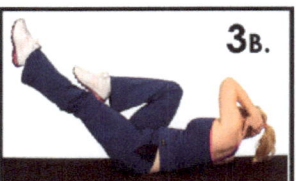

3B.

Advanced 3B.

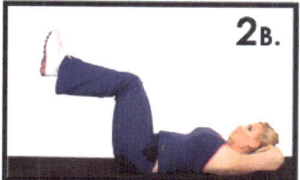

2. Core Heel Tap

Begin lying on your back with your knees bent 90 degrees and chins parallel to the ground. Hands should be in back of your head. Begin with an inhale and engage the abs, but pulling them in towards the spine. On the exhale lower your right heel to lightly touch the ground. On the inhale bring it back to the start position. Repeat on the other side. This should be done as a slow and controlled movement for 20 reps on each side.

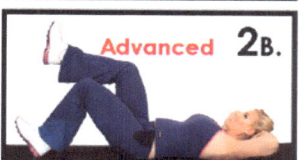

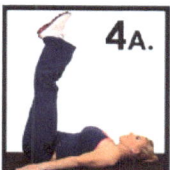

4. Hip Lift

Begin lying on your back with your knees bent 90 degrees and chins Begin lying flat on the back with the legs straight, toes elevated to the ceiling and above the hips. This is a small movement. On the exhale lift the hips off the ground about 2-4 inches, enough to feel the tailbone come off the ground. This movement will engage the lower abdominals first. A key to remember is not to let the feet swing to lift the feet up. You want to keep your toes as much over your hips as possible. Repeat this movement for 20 reps.

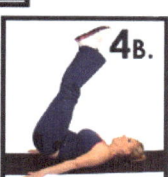

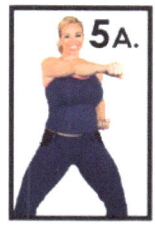

5. Torso Punch

Stand with your feet about 2-3 feet apart with the toes turned out about 45 degrees and the knees slightly bent. Place both fists on your hips with the palms facing upwards and elbows pointing to the rear. By engaging your internal and external obliques begin rotating the upper body only. Extend the right arm horizontally across the body to the left with the hand in a fist and palm facing down. Squeeze the back of the extended arm to get triceps flexion. Repeat on the other side. Keep the head looking straight ahead at all times. Perform this exercise for 20-50 reps on each side.

These five exercises can be repeated for three sets of each or you can rotate through all five exercises and repeat the series three times. Really focus on the coordination of the breathing and most importantly engaging the abs by keeping them pulled in towards the spine during each movement.

A "congratulations" to you if you have just had your baby and you are now getting back into your exercise groove. This is also a perfect routine if you have taken a break from exercising for a period of time. Regardless of where you are physically, this is a safe and gradual way to increase your abdominal and core strength.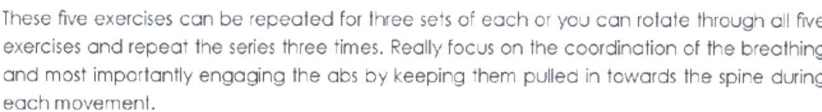

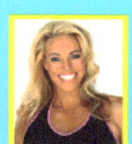

ABOUT THE WRITER: Over the past 19 years Laura Mak has made it part of her career in fitness to be a leader, a forward thinker, and a positive role model in every way when she undertakes a new project. Since her early days in training as an elite athlete and then on to the top ranks as an *IFBB Fitness Pro*, Laura Mak has taken her passion for Lifestyle Fitness Coaching to a level only reached by the top echelon in the fitness industry.

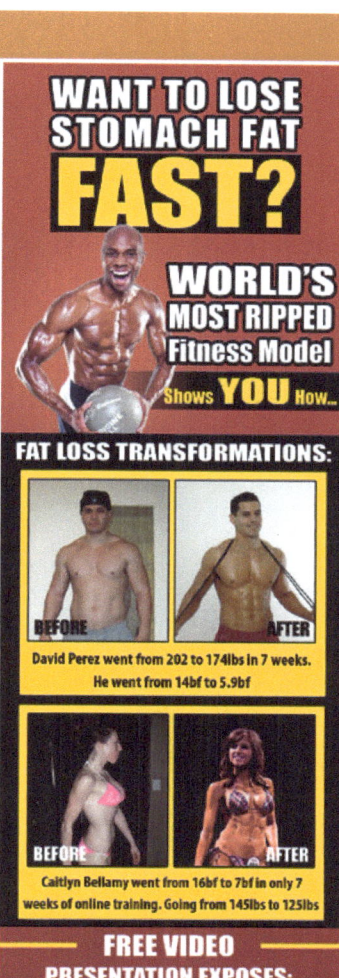
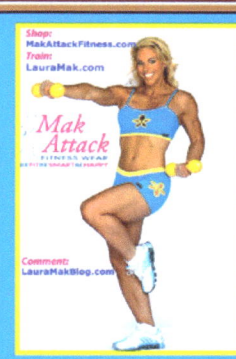

What *Forever* Changed Me

WRITTEN BY: Chandra Whitaker Cobb

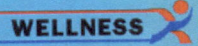

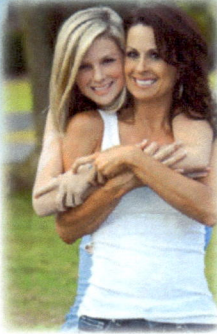

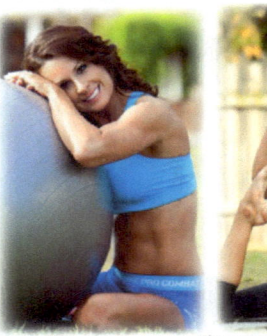
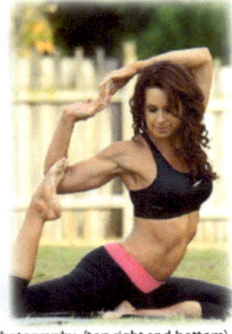

BEFORE Snapshot by family friend

AFTER Photos by: Raw Images Photography (top right and bottom)

My name is Chandra Whitaker Cobb. I am 39-year-old wife and mother of two amazing children. Born and raised in the small town of Hanceville, Alabama, I have to admit finding myself writing this story is something that I never imagined would be possible. Then again, I also never imagined I would have a weight gain of 50 pounds either.

Up until four years ago, I was extremely active in my local gym and very fit, but on August 6, 2007 my life took a drastic change. My husband had just changed jobs, moved our family across state and was in the process of buying a new home. And, as if that's not enough stress, the next event changed my life forever.

My two children were in a tragic golf cart accident. I remember that day as if it were yesterday. My husband brought the cart home on his lunch that was an early birthday gift for our daughter. She was on top of the world, but oh how fast that all changed. One moment, they are passing in front of the house singing as those rode laps around the neighborhood, and the next she severely scratched. Little did I know until I reached for her how brutal the accident had been. At this time, Reagan was 8 and her younger brother was just 2. The babysitter was driving the cart when she accidentally lost control and flipped it...slamming Reagan on the asphalt and dragging her 55 feet under the cart down a steep hill, with Reese and the older child on top of her. After the was walking through the door covered in blood and holding her arm, which at the time appeared to be golf cart stopped, all the children, only by the grace of God, gathered themselves and walked two blocks back up the hill they had just slid down to the house.

Everything was happening so fast-- the baby was crying which was also covered in blood, Reagan was passing out and the babysitter was still in shock. After calling 911, a person who till this day I refer to as my angel, appeared out of nowhere and assisted me with all three children until the paramedics arrived, and just like she appeared, disappeared without saying a word. Reagan was then swept away in air flight to the hospital, leaving me not knowing if I would ever see her again.

The drive was long, but after arriving at the hospital, we found that Reese had a broken collar bone. The head injury Reagan had sustained was minor, but her arm wasn't. Her right arm was dragged under the golf cart, snapping it and eroding all bone and muscle tissue. We were told if she kept the arm, which was basically amputated, she would never use it again because of all the nerve and muscle damage. So, with 8 days in the hospital and two major surgeries later, my focus was on my children and not my nutrition or workouts this is where let go of myself and the weight gain began.

See what I mean, when I talk about life changing? It's times like these when we are forced beyond our control to change our direction. Mine was no longer on health or fitness, but on the well being of my children.

Now jump forward with me -- February 2010 -- Reagan and Reese both fully recovered and are thriving, however, I was not doing so well. Now I find myself larger than I have ever been in my life and extremely unhappy about myself image. My weight gain didn't happen overnight, (it never does), but 2lbs here and 3lbs there start to add up. Watching "Biggest Loser" one Tuesday night with my children, I looked at my daughter and said "I want to be Jillian Michaels." She said, "Mom, you can do It!" So, the next day I began my fitness journey.

I remember walking into that gym embarrassed and scared but determined. I took a Les Mills class *BODYPUMP* with this amazing instructor Brooke Nicole who was so motivating. She kicked my butt, but surprisingly I wanted more. She came to me after class and complimented me on my form, and that's all it took, I was hooked. I didn't miss a class and the weight slowly started coming off, but I couldn't help but want more. So In April 2010 I attended a *Les Mills* training weekend and became certified to teach YOGA. Always having wanted to teach, but never having the courage I was living a dream and all it took was someone believing in me. The year rocked on still losing a pound here and there but still missing something...Then the day came in February 2011, almost one year from my start date, I received a text from Brooke Nicole. All it said was " *Southern Classic NPC in June*", and I was in...

As some say "GAME ON!" In March, I hired my first trainer, David Leveritt, owner of Fitness South in Tuscaloosa, Alabama to help prepare me for my bikini competition in June. Shortly following the show in June, I joined Cathy Savage Fitness (CSF); I can just say this lady has changed my life forever. I competed in two more shows this past year finishing 2nd in both.

Today, I am a Certified Personal Trainer and Group Fitness Instructor. Through CSF, I maintain a healthy nutrition and exercise program closely monitored by my personal coach. My goal as a trainer is to let women know that we may have those unexpected occurrences in our life that can cause us to lose ourselves, but don't give up and think you are alone.

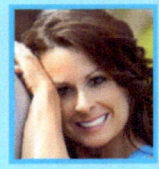

Chandra Whitaker Cobb is a 39-year-old wife and mother of two children, turned fitness competitor, model and trainer. She was born and raised in the small town of Hanceville, Alabama. Growing up, Chandra was always involved in dance, cheerleading and gymnastics which carried over into her college years. After graduating and even marriage, Chandra was able to maintain her health and fitness until the summer of 2007. This is when her life changed forever. Currently, Chandra resides in Guntersville, Alabama and spends her time teaching yoga, bootcamp and personal training women of all ages at Power House Gym in Albertville, AL and Flex Fitness in Arab, AL helping others overcome the same struggles she dealt with herself just a year ago.

You have to "BELIEVE TO ACHIEVE"!
Follow your dreams and know that
there is someone out there
who believes in you.
For me, it was (and still is today),
my Savage Sister, Brooke Nicole.

CORE - Center of your Existence - Your Inner Existence is God

WRITTEN BY: Sherry Goggin
PHOTO BY: BillyBow Photography

What is the center of your life and the ground of your existence?

When you close your eyes, you can reflect upon the inner nature and you become the observer of everything inside you. When you try to observe the observer, you will touch the pure existence, which is the image of God, which has all the perfections of God.

Existence everywhere is one and it is God. It is reality. It is that which sustains our life and all of our experiences, all our knowing and feeling. Without existence we are nothing and without God we are nothing.

The real source of being happy is not amidst our thoughts or possessions, not in the senses of the body. It is only there in the existence which is all pure. As you know, your thoughts come and go. They may cause some kind of happiness which is temporary, as it will quickly disappear. The disappearances causes unhappiness.

The presence of God is everywhere and it is all-knowing, all-observing, all consciousness and all beauty, all freedom, all light, all harmony, all wealth and all power.

The more you reflect upon this central reality, the greater and stronger your knowledge of that central reality becomes and you will arrive at that which is the source of endless happiness and endless life – (eternal life through Jesus). -John 3:16

"For God loved the world so much that he gave his one and only Son, so that everyone who believes in him will not perish but have eternal life."

OVERCOME every situation in Life?

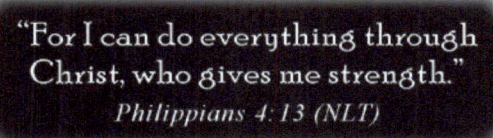

"For I can do everything through Christ, who gives me strength."
Philippians 4:13 (NLT)

There is no set back in life that you can face that God doesn't already have a comeback plan for you.

Some people will overcome their mistakes and move on to the greater things God has in store for them. Unfortunately, some people just can't do that. God has created you to be an overcomer and he wants and will lift you up!

The Apostle Paul writes in Romans: "Don't copy the behavior and customs of this world, but let God transform you into a new person by changing the way you think. Then you will learn to know God's will for you, which is good and pleasing and perfect" (Romans 12:2 NLT).

All you have to do is let this new attitude FORM your thinking and God will lift you up out of your current circumstances and bring you into the amazing purposes that God has planned for you.

CHANGE YOUR THINKING AND TRANSFORM YOUR LIFE!

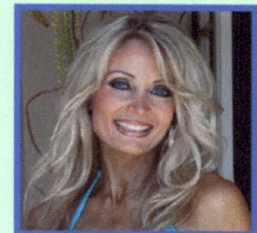

ABOUT THE WRITER: Sherry Goggin, Ms. Fitness America, reigns as The Most Photographed Fitness model in history. She shines as author, producer and role model for women everywhere. Bright, articulate and full of energy, Goggin has broken the stereotype of the fitness model to become an author, producer, fitness guru, clothes designer and just about anything else she puts her mind to. Sherry Goggin is the definitive version of a 'renaissance woman' and once she sets her mind to something, nothing gets in her way. And right now, she has her mind set on being a success. While Goggin is a fitness expert, her real strengths may lie in the area of being a top-notch business entrepreneur. She also acts as VP and director of the women's fitness division of the Private Trainers association, www.propta.com. Sherry also has a new clothing line, "Fit Girl Wear" that is available for purchase now. All of Sherry's merchandise is available for purchase at any of her websites including www.SherryGoggin.com, facebook.com/sherrygoggin and modelmayhem.com/sherrygoggin. Photo by: BillyBow Photography

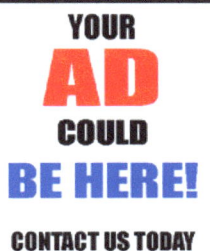

FITNESS X
APPAREL STORE
Get your fitness
& fashion gear!
http://www.cafepress.com/fitnessx
FITNESS INSPIRING
FITNESS INSPIRING
FITNESS
FITNESS HEALTH - FITNESS - WELLNESS Magazine
FITNESS HEALTH - FITNESS - WELLNESS Magazine
FITNESS INSPIRING
SIGG
FITNESS INSPIRING

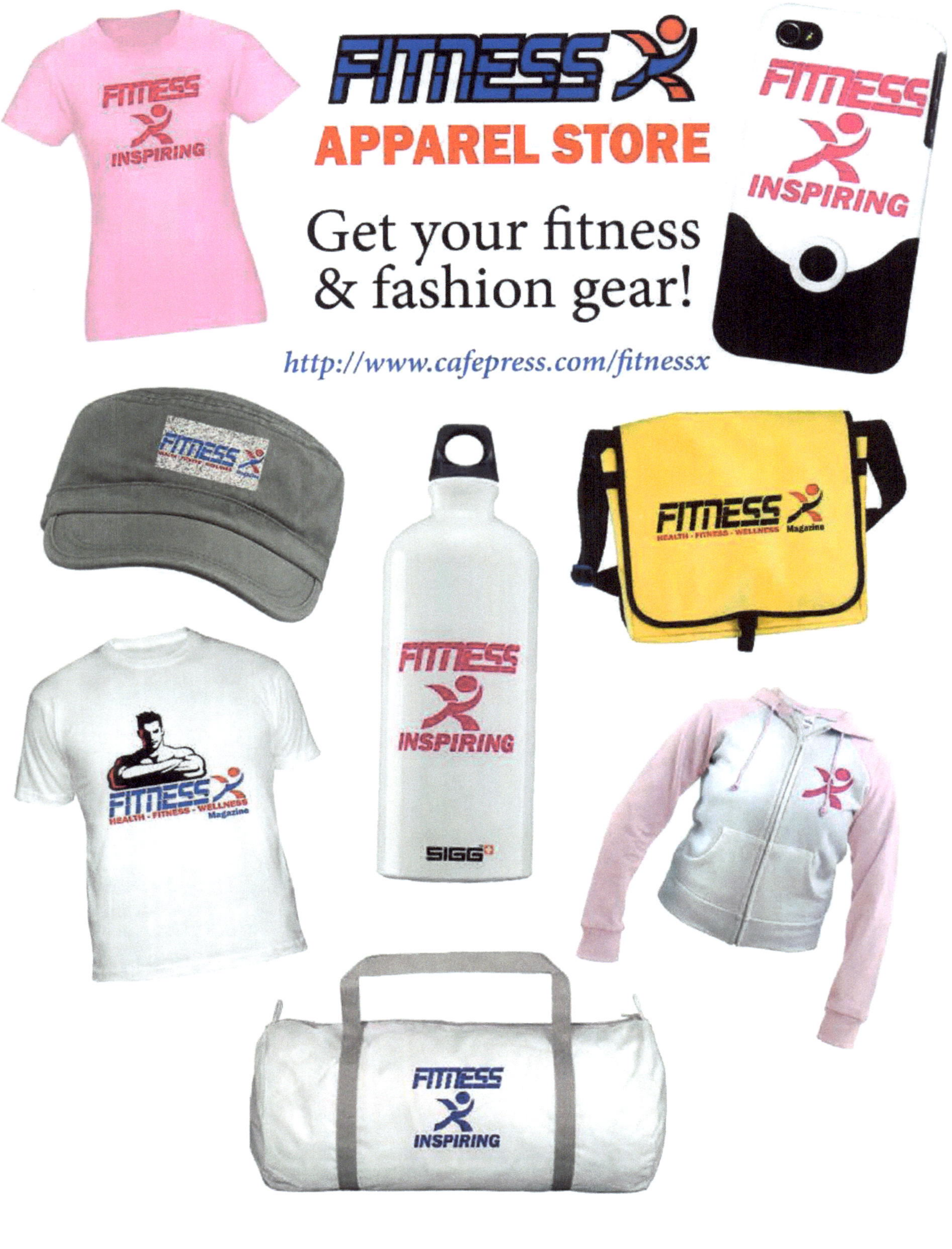

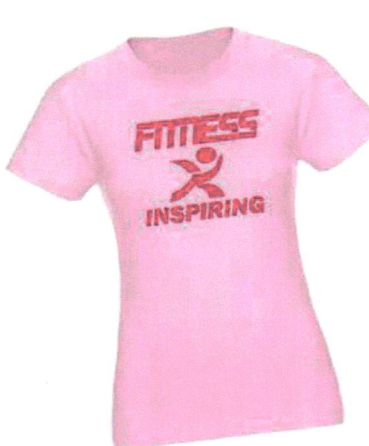

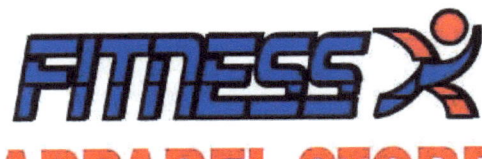

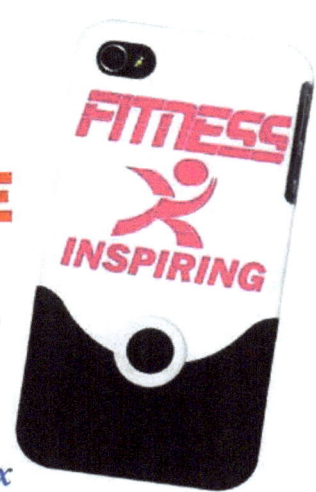

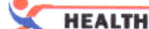
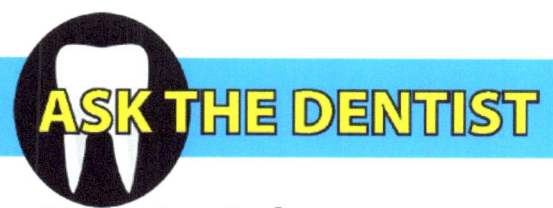

ASK THE DENTIST

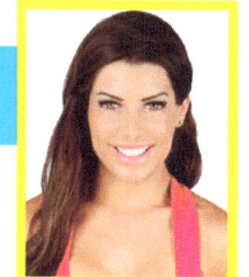

Dear Dr. Solomon,

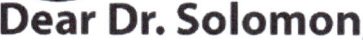

Q = **I've been hearing about health risks associated with water fluoridation. Is this true?"**

What is fluoridated water?

Fluoride is a naturally occurring mineral that is scientifically proven to protect against tooth decay. Fluoride prevents tooth decay by slowing the activity of bacteria that cause decay and by combining with tooth enamel to make it stronger and more resistant to decay. Almost all water contains naturally occurring fluoride; however, this naturally occurring fluoride is not present in sufficient levels to prevent tooth decay. Fluoridation of community water is simply the adjustment of this pre-existing fluoride level to a higher level of 0.7 parts per million (ppm) as recommended by the U.S. Department of Health and Human Services (HHS) to prevent tooth decay. This value of 0.7ppm (0.7 mg of fluoride per liter of water) has recently replaced the previous range of 0.7 to 1.2 ppm that was originally recommended in 1962 by the U.S Public Health Service.

Why the change?

Sources of fluoride exposure have increased since 1962. In the 1960s, the only source of fluoride exposure was from drinking fluoridated water. Today, we are also exposed to fluoride in the form of toothpaste, mouthwash, topical fluoride treatments at the dental office and prescription fluoride supplements. Thanks to these advances, even with a slightly lower level of fluoride in water, you will still receive enough fluoride to reduce your risk of tooth decay. To learn if your community has fluoridated water, you can call your public water system.

Why 0.7ppm?

The level 0.7ppm is recommended because it provides the benefits of preventing tooth decay while minimizing the risk of dental fluorosis. Dental fluorosis appears as white spots on the teeth, which does not pose any danger to health: it is merely a cosmetic concern. Dental fluorosis results when children regularly consume higher than the recommended amounts of fluoride during the years when their teeth are forming (≤8 years of age). If your child is exclusively consuming infant formula reconstituted with fluoridated water, there may be an increased chance for mild dental fluorosis. Lessen this chance by using low-fluoride bottled water some of the time, rather than using fluoridated water exclusively.

What are the adverse effects of excessive fluoride exposure?

As we previously stated, excessive exposure to fluoride impacts teeth while they are forming. This can occur anytime from birth to 8 years of age. If children in this age group are exposed to excessive amounts of fluoride, then they have an increased chance of developing pits and other un-aesthetic effects on their teeth. To minimize the risk of unsightly fluorosis from excessive fluoride consumption, do not let your child start using fluoridated toothpaste until he/she is 2 years old and able to spit out the excess toothpaste. Fluoride toothpaste does not contribute to fluorosis unless it is swallowed. Only use a pea-sized amount on the brush and ensure your child can rinse well after spitting. Supervise your child's oral hygiene regime until he/she is 6 years of age. Children under 6 years of age must not be given fluoridated mouthwashes, as they may swallow it.
If adults are exposed to excessive long-term fluoride consumption, they have an increased risk of bone fractures and skeletal fluorosis. Skeletal fluorosis presents as bone pain and tenderness. This is a rare condition in the United States. Those at greatest risk live in areas with high natural background levels of fluoride. Remember that some regions in the United States have naturally high levels of fluoride in the drinking water. In the event that your home is served by a water system that has fluoride levels exceeding 2.0 ppm, then it is recommended to use an alternative source of drinking water.

Is fluoridate water safe?

The American Dental Association supports community water fluoridation as a "safe, beneficial and cost-effective way to prevent tooth decay". Peer-reviewed scientific evidence does not support an association between water fluoridation and any adverse health effect or systemic disorders. The Centers for Disease Control and Prevention (CDC) has proclaimed community water fluoridation as one of the 10 great public health achievements of the 20th century. ✗

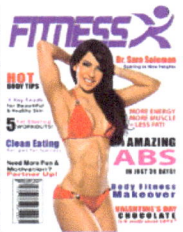

ABOUT THE WRITER: Dr. Sara Solomon received her BSc in Physical Therapy and her DMD from McGill University in 2001 and 2005 respectively. She is a general dentist in Toronto, Ontario, Canada. Sara is also a WBFF PRO Fitness Model, a writer, a cover girl, a certified personal trainer, a SPINNING® instructor, a physiotherapist, a certified jump rope specialist with the Jump Rope Institute, a university and continuing education lecturer and a photographer. To learn more about Sara, please visit her website at www.drsarasolomon.com. E-mail your questions for Dr. Solomon to publisher@fitnessX. com

I am a COMPETITOR... a SURVIVOR!

Written by: Alyssian Vissat

Photo by: Capturesque Photography

Many of us are told we have our whole lives ahead of us, but what may come as a surprise is we don't. At any moment, someone or something can divert us away from our dearest dreams and aspirations. We soon find life is full of intersections and it's how we handle them that get us through. In one split second, a determined, young woman would stumble onto such an intersection. She would have to make sacrifices, endure pains, watch her body deteriorate, and find strengths she never knew she had.

Crystal Bragazzi, now a 30-year old woman, grew up in Littleton, Colorado. "Growing up, I always wanted to become a police officer." At 23 years old, she started working as a case manager and continuing to train for the police academy. Crystal stated, "I was in excellent shape. Probably the best shape ever." In May 2004, she was accepted into the Lakewood Police Academy commencing later in August. Crystal was getting excited when Lakewood Police Department (L.P.D.) called June 1st to inform her for a second time, they could not afford to have a police academy. "I was devastated ... and fed up."

Her next journey would be with Las Vegas Metro; but, to her dismay, she awoke June 7, 2004 to a tender and swollen left side of her neck. She assumed it was a strained muscle. A couple days went by when her mother demanded Crystal see a doctor. On June 11th, she visited her doctor explaining how she wanted to continue her training but not cause anymore damage to the assumed strained muscle. The doctor briefly felt her neck and informed Crystal, "That's not a muscle. It's a lymphoid ... you have cancer!" At that moment, Crystal was not too sure what to think but her face looked as if she had seen a ghost. She scheduled the next step, a needle biopsy.

Four days later, the doctors' drained fluid from her lymphoid as well as scheduled a surgical biopsy. The fluid tested positive for cancer and three days after her needle biopsy, Crystal would have the biopsy to type the cancer. When it comes to lymphoma, there are two types, Hodgkin's and Non-Hodgkin's. Hodgkin's is known if caught early, to be easier to treat and chances of it coming back are less than that of Non-Hodgkin's. Crystal soon found ways to keep her mind off what she was about to face.

Crystal still planned on testing with Las Vegas Metro. She stepped up her training; pushing her self farther and harder each day. After all, a girl with cancer could not run like she could. Crystal flew to Las Vegas putting her treatment on hold. Returning home was the last thing she wanted to do. July 8th was her first appointment with the oncologist where she was told she did have Hodgkin's. It spread from her neck into her chest and treatment would be aggressive with chemotherapy and radiation. Crystal was determined not to let cancer get the best of her training. That same day, Crystal took her first steps into the chemo room.

Crystal would spend 4 hours in a room every other week until December 10th, 2004. "The worst part about chemo was how I felt after. It literally felt like someone had kicked my butt. . . . my whole body hurt. Food tasted horrible. I had trouble breathing." It was after the first treatment Crystal realized training was out of the question. She would have to find other ways to stay active. She bought a dog to take on walks and named her "Kima" inspired after reading Lance Armstrong's It's Not about the Bike. Crystal ended up in the hospital twice, gained over 25 pounds, had to give herself daily injections, and started to lose her hair. Crystal spent the mornings cleaning up her hair and eventually decided to shave it. Crystal and her father shaved each other's heads. "This was a moment I will never forget." Crystal endured 30 days of radiation treatment as well as brea "I had nothing to lose and everything to gain, so I made a commitment to get back in shape, lose the weight, and compete." st surgery.

The radiation burned her throat and skin. Eating became intolerable. She lost 25 pounds in two weeks and forced herself to drink protein shakes and water. Her last day of treatments and first day of remission was February 17th, 2005. A month later, she was hired onto L.P.D. where she worked for 6 years as a beat cop, undercover, and a detective in the major crimes unit. Four years into her dream job, she went in for breast surgery. "I was at the lowest point in my life... I let myself go." Crystal soon realized just how hard it was to get her body back to where it once was, but she was up for the challenge.

On June of 2011, she started as a Probation Officer as well as began to reignite her passion for staying in

> "I had nothing to lose and **EVERYTHING** to **GAIN**, so I made a **COMMITMENT** to get back in shape, lose the weight, & compete."

Model: Crystal Bragazzi

shape. This job gave her more time to spend in "The Gym" where two of her friends were training to compete in local bikini competitions. "I had nothing to lose and everything to gain, so I made a commitment to get back in shape, lose the weight, and compete." Crystal took stage in November with the constant support of her family and team members, "The Miss Fits". She lost over 20 lbs. and looks forward to competing again this year. We don't have forever to live; but when life's intersections hand us challenges, it is our choice on how we handle them. It is our choice to accept them. It is our choice to push through the pains and see what parts of ourselves we are willing to sacrifice to get through. Some intersections are easier than others. We can only hope for the best and continue to fight for our dreams and hopes as Crystal continues to do.

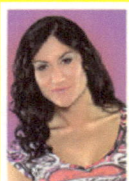
Alyssian Vissat has been active ever since she can remember. She was a varsity cheerleader for two years in high school, a semi-pro cheerleader for the CFC, a pro cheerleader for the IFL, go-go danced for many events, modeled for the last 10+ years, and travelled with a race team where she was not only an umbrella girl & spokesmodel, she was part of the pit crew, and all of the opportunities led her to her training facility, The Gym which also inspired her to start her own unique clothing line (www.tophercouture.com). She started training at The Gym in 2007, but took her four years to finally take stage in the 2011 NPC Colorado Natural. The Gym's fitness team, "The Miss Fits", had finally taken form and inspired Aly to get on stage. A group of dedicated, beautiful, motivating women had entered and changed her life along with God's help. Alyssian was inspired by her fellow teammate's story. She lost her father when she was 14 years old to Non-Hodgkin's Lymphoma. She hopes Crystal's story will inspire others, who have suffered and are suffering, to have hope. Each breath taken is a blessing! Photo by: Capturesque Photography · www.capturesque.com

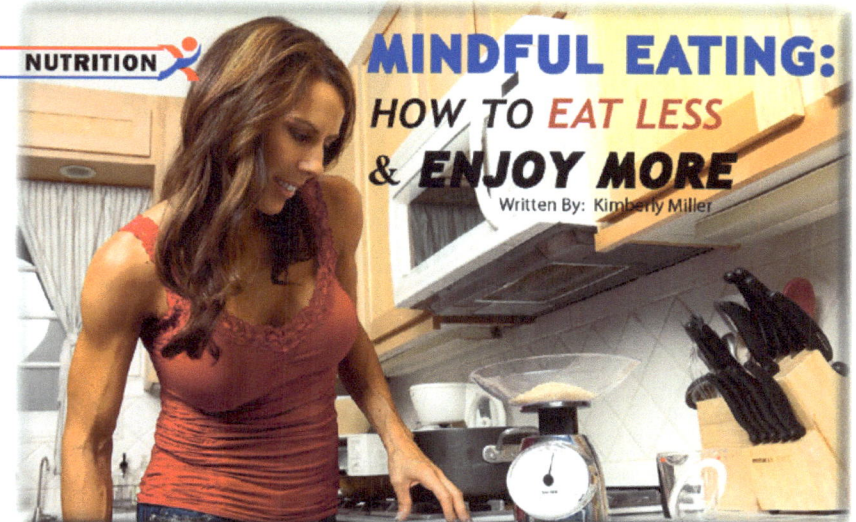

MINDFUL EATING:
HOW TO EAT LESS & ENJOY MORE
Written By: Kimberly Miller

Leha Long's Recipe
BREAKFAST BURRITO

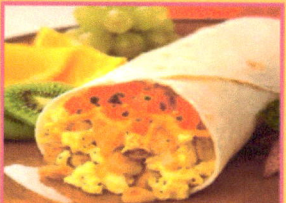

Short of time for cooking? No need to stress! Here's a few quick and easy recipes you can put together fast! Here are a few of my favorite wrap recipes that includes low carbs, lean protein, and healthy fats. Remember to cook ahead of time to keep you from eating unhealthy food! (1 Burrito = 315 Calories)

Ingredients:

- . 1 Low-Carb Low-Fat Soft Taco Tortilla
- · 6 tbsp. Liquid Egg Whites
- · 2.5 oz Extra Lean Ground Turkey Breast
- · 1/4 cup Onions, Raw
- · 1/4 cup of Avocados, Raw
- · 1/3 cup Sliced Green Peppers

Directions:

Cook the turkey, onions, avocado, and bell peppers. Scramble the eggwhites in a pan that has been sprayed with cooking spray. Remove the eggs, then spray the pan again and place the tortilla in the pan. While the tortilla is cooking, place the scrambled eggs, chopped onions, green peppers, and turkey on top. Wrap the tortilla around the mix and enjoy!

What happens when you're hungry? You find the quickest and most convenient thing you can get your hands on and eat it. This pattern is definitely something many individuals have to retrain themselves on when they set goals for improving their health and losing weight. The goal becomes to avoid finding yourself in a position where you are over-hungry, especially in the presence of a fast food restaurant!

What is mindful eating anyway, and how can it help you achieve your goals? According to The Center for Mindful (TCME), "It's allowing yourself to become aware of the positive and nurturing opportunities that are available through food preparation and consumption by respecting your own inner wisdom." What does that mean? It's about fully enjoying the process of eating and paying careful attention to what food does to your body. In an effort to ensure you are being mindful of your eating habits, consider trying the following tips when nourishing yourself.

Mindful Eating for Meal Time:

1) Prepare meals and snacks in advance: Rather than just grabbing food on the go, prepping for meals allows you to develop a keener sense of your body, how to care for your health, and how to appreciate and respect food. Doing this allows you to fully recognize the quantities you consume, the type of foods you are drawn to, and the process whereby foods are cooked. Relaying on others to prepare the items you consume releases your control of knowing what you are putting in your body. Look through cook books, find recipes or ideas, and subscribe to blogs or sites on food that give suggestions. Shop local farmers markets and talk to the growers. Think carefully about what goes into growing food and pay particular

2) Allocate time to prepare meals and eat together: Slowing down makes you more appreciative of what you are putting in your body. Even the art of buying bags of almonds and portioning them out makes you more aware of how much a serving is, what it offers you nutritionally, and how filling it is. When creating meals for your family, concentrate on the entire process from food preparation to consumption. Make eating an experience rather than just an act.

3) Savor the moment: When you sit down at the table, close your eyes for a moment. Think about what you are about to ingest and how it will nourish your body. Are you eating empty calories? If so, that's oaky, just be aware. Does your plate have the variety of colors on it? Is the food on your plate a blend of the vital nutrients you need to sustain yourself. Take a moment to truly think about what you are eating. Being in the moment allows you to more carefully decide when you are still hungry and eating for nourishment and when you are indulging.

4) Make eating a ritual : Start by having a glass of water to cleanse the palate. Ensure you are not going into meals over-hungry. Breathe deeply and smell the aroma of the food. As you eat, pay aattention to the different flavors. Eat slowly and intentionally. Pause between bites to allow your body time to take in the flavors and textures. This will ensure you don't overeat. Before you reach for a second helping, give your body time to digest.

5) Reflect: After eating, notice how your body reacts. Did the foods you ingest make you feel good and give you energy, or did they take away from those things? Many people have food allergies or sensitivities, and go years before they ever realize it. Everyone is different. You are the best judge of knowing what food works for you! Some people avoid dairy, others avoid red meat; some are vegetarians and others vegan; some can't have gluten and some have sugar intolerance. You are the owner of your body. Only you know what makes you feel good. Pay attention to your body and figure this out.

Most importantly, remember that mindful eating is not prescribing to a specific diet plan. According to Dr. Susan Albers of the Cleveland Clinic Family Health Center, a specialist in eating issues who conducts workshops around the globe, mindful eating is, "being more aware of your eating habits, the sensations you experience when you eat, and the thoughts and emotions that you have about food. It's more about how you eat then what you eat." Eating right and caring for yourself is a skill. Feed the body good whole foods, appreciate the moments of eating, pay careful attention to the process, love yourself, share your successes and tips, learn from your failures, and support others. This will go a long way toward achieving your goals for optimum health. ✗

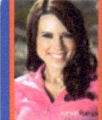

Kim Miller works in the talent industry as is a Stylist, Fitness Motivator, Writer, and Commercial & Fitness Talent. It was during her graduate work at Miami University where her love of writing developed and she produces articles not only related to her passions, but also on genuineness and realness.Kim's fitness articles are featured on the *Arizona Republic Newspaper*'s site www.azcvoices.com and her recent fitness styling work can be seen on the January cover of *Scottsdale Health Magazine*. She is currently an official candidate for the Mrs. Arizona America Pageant and an active fitness and commercial talent. Her podcast, *The ProExposure* (www.theproexposure.com), seeks to help educate people in the Fitness and Talent Industry. Kim Miller's blog can be viewed at www.TheModernMe.wordpress.com. Photo credit: James Patrick

GEO
Gifted Earth Originals

GEO Organic Egg White Protein Powder

We choose to raise our chickens without cages and with access to the outdoors so our flocks are able to live naturally and gift back to us very high quality eggs. We promote Family Farms and Humane-Raised livestock practices. We believe our Earth will continue to provide its gifts to us now and in the future if we respect it and make good choices.

Try the world's first organic egg white protein powder in flavors such as: Very Strawberry, Chocolate Divine and Vibrant Vanilla. Also comes in Plain. Enjoy the rich smoothness and sweet taste.

Gifted Earth Originals is great for:
- Strength and conditioning training
- Managing weight
- Low cholesterol diets
- Ovo-vegetarian diets
- Gluten-free

GEO SPONSORED ATHLETE
Keri Lynn Ford

photo by: Eva Simon

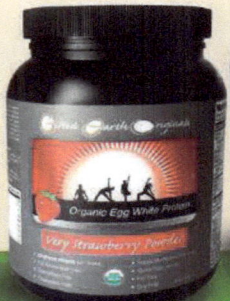
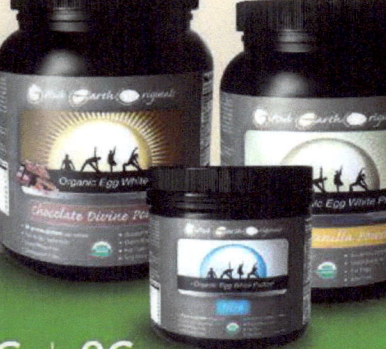

100% ORGANIC | **25G** PROTEIN | **0G** FAT

Available at
amazon.com

For more information, facts or recipes
visit giftedearthoriginals.com

Keri Ford's Recipe
GEO Trail Mix
Protein Brownies

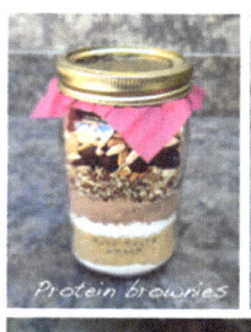
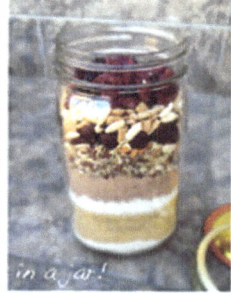

Protein brownies in a jar!

Layer Dry Ingredients in Jar:

- Layer 1: 1/2 cup oat flour, 1/4 teaspoon baking powder, 1/4 teaspoon salt
- Layer 2: 1 cup raw turbinado sugar
- Layer 3: 1/2 cup organic shredded coconut
- Layer 4: 1/3 cup unsweetened dark cocoa powder mixed with 4 scoops GEO Chocolate Divine Protein Powder
- Layer 5: chopped, mixed nuts (pecans, walnuts, almonds)
- Layer 6: 1/3 cup dark chocolate chips
- Layer 7: 1/3 cup Kashi cereal or chopped pretzels
- Layer 8: 1/4 cup dried cranberries or raisins

Simply add wet ingredients when you are ready to bake:

- 2 teaspoons vanilla extract
- 1/3 cup olive oil
- 3 large egg whites
- 2 large whole eggs
- PAM

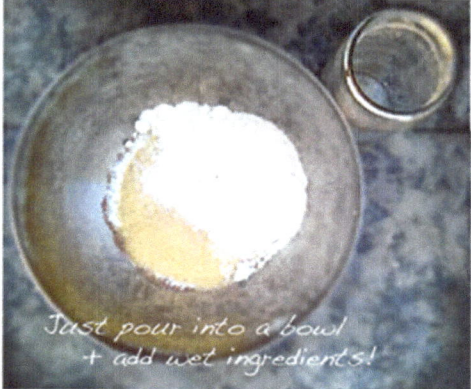

Just pour into a bowl + add wet ingredients!

Layer dry ingredients into a mason jar and give as a gift! (label with a handmade tag with instructions on how to bake below)

Preheat oven to 350º F. Spray an 8" by 8" metal baking pan with PAM. Pour jar contents into large bowl.

In a small bowl, whisk oil, vanilla, and eggs until well mixed, then pour into large bowl to blend with oat flour mixture.

Spread in greased pan.

Sprinkle top with mixed trail mix (chopped pretzels, shredded coconut, mixed nuts, dried cranberries, chocolate chips) halfway through.

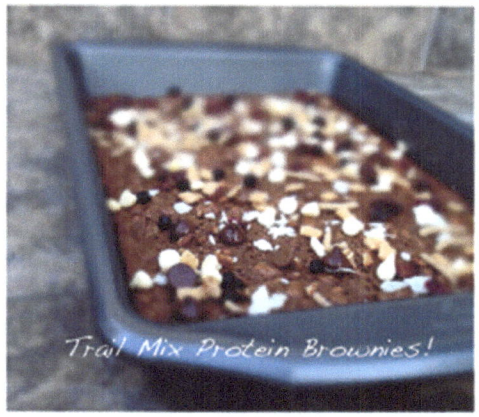

Trail Mix Protein Brownies!

Bake 22 to 24 minutes or until toothpick inserted in brownies a couples inches from edge comes out almost clean.

Cool in pan on wire rack for about two hours. When cool, cut brownies into squares and serve.

* Try dipping a knife in hot water, wipe dry and cut if browies are difficult to cut. Repeat as necessary.

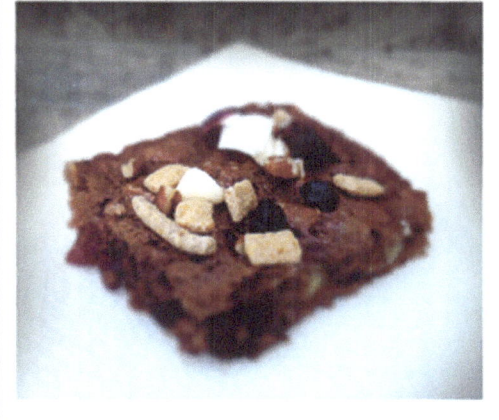

6 Steps to Your 6-Pack!

WRITTEN BY: Vince Delmonte

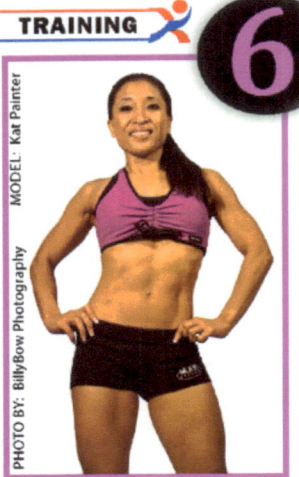

MODEL: Kat Painter

PHOTO BY: BillyBow Photography

Don't get fooled and fall for the hype. Getting a midsection that sets you apart from the pack requires the traits of practicality and patience. Ripped six-pack abs – the ones that cause jealousy – are unquestionably the most desired visual benefit of hard-training fitness enthusiasts. Sure, it's impressive to have sculpted legs, firm arms, or flat abs, but most practical gym-goers are seeking out visual impact from head to toe. A swimsuit doesn't look aesthesically pleasing when it's intersected with a big, bulging stomach. Got abs? Now you own the trophy of all trophies!

Rule #1: Cut Your Calories By 20%

On average, most individuals consume about 17 calories per pound of bodyweight each day. It's important to cut back the amount of food you're eating to create a slight caloric deficit, encouraging your body to tap into body fat for energy to make up the difference. Most individuals should reduce their overall calorie consumption about 20% during the first two weeks, taking in about 14 calories per pound of body weight each day. For example, if you weigh 200 lbs., you should be eating around 2,800 calories a day (200 x 14 = 2,800). You can reduce your calories another 20%, if you're not losing at least 1% of your body weight per week.

Rule #2: Eat Five Solid Meals & One Shake

Establishing a regular meal cadence of five solid meals a day, rather than 3 meals a day, helps your body experience a slight increase in calorie-burning. Every time you eat, your body uses energy (calories) to break down, digest, and absorb the food you eat. Consuming multiple meals helps lower cortisol levels (a catabolic hormone), which results in slightly elevated testosterone levels (a muscle-building hormone). The higher your testosterone levels, the greater your muscle growth and more muscle leads to more calorie burning. My mantra: "Eat solid food if you want to look solid." Immediately after an intense workout, consume a liquid meal consisting of fast-acting proteins and carbs in the form of whey-isolate and carb powder such at Karbolyn, Vtargo, maltodextrin, dextrose, or Gatorade. We consume fluids after our workout because the nutrients are delivered faster than whole food.

Rule #3: It's Paramount You Eat "Clean" Carbohydrates

Not all carbs are created equal (too bad)! In fact, many "natural" carbs are fast-digesting (glucose/sugar-based). When you consume this type of carb, they trigger an insulin spike that encourages bodyfat storage. Instead, slow-digesting carbs are better because they reduce your insulin response – they will also stay with you longer, preventing hunger pains, controlling appetite, and preventing crashing during your workouts. Carbs will also give your physique a full, strong, and healthy appearance – not a weak and soft look. Consume in the form of a slow-digesting, long-lasting carb like oatmeal, brown rice, Ezekiel cereal, quinoa, whole-wheat breads or pastas, whole fruits, yams, sweet-potatoes, and whole vegetables such as broccoli, spinach, asparagus, and squash. In addition to recommendations above, include high-fiber foods such as beans and lentils, as well as low-fructose fruits. Your carb intake should be approximately 40% of your daily intake starting out, and can be adjusted up or down slightly, based on the speed of your metabolism.

Rule #4: Be Deserving Of Your Carbohydrates

Carbohydrates are not the enemy when it comes to burning fat: too many calories and low- quality food is the enemy. Time your carbohydrates around the times of the day you deserve them – 1 to 1.5 hours before you workout, immediately after your workout, one hour after you workout, and 4 hours after you workout. This carbohydrate timing strategy will ensure you refuel your muscle glycogen stores and have plenty in reserve for your daily tasks.

Rule #5: Bump Up Your Protein Intake

Consuming 1 to 1.5 grams of protein per pound of bodyweight every day, spread out through the day, is your goal. This works out to approximately 40% of your daily caloric intake. Ensure your protein comes in a variety of sources to optimize digestion and absorption. By providing a steady stream of amino acids, you're supplying your muscles with a buffer to prevent breakdown. These aminos will be used for physiological processes, and your body is much less likely to break down muscle tissue for use of energy, which can occur as you get ultra lean. Maintaining a high protein diet helps increase your metabolic rate, meaning your body needs more calories just to maintain its bodyweight. The best news is that this also makes it easier for your body to burn fat. For optimal results, avoid eating the same protein source more than once a day. Strive to eat at least 6 different sources of protein each day. You can include different types of white fish such as cod, haddock, sea bass, halibut, flounder, tilapia, sole, and turbot. When it comes to meat, try to rotate bison, buffalo patties, chicken, lean beef, elk, ostrich, venison, wild boar, turkey, kangaroo, and even antelope (many of these meats can be found in exotic meat stores). Finally, including egg whites, cottage cheese, whole eggs, and whey-isolate protein will ensure you never experience diet boredom!

Rule #6: Eat More Fat To Burn Fat

A huge mistake is going too low with your fat intake. You need to consume a certain amount of dietary fat for satiety (making you feel full), hormone production, and general sense of well-being. Strive to get at least 20% of your daily calories from fat. Consider fat your "happy" food – cut your fat and you'll feel like a truck ran over you. When it comes to fat selection, the rule is the same as proteins and fats: variety is key. Find a balance between a few great oils to receive the benefits of each. Macadamia oil, olive oil, and coconut oil are excellent. Include whole food sources such as walnuts, cashews, almonds, pecans, and avocados. To optimize hormones, it's best to never consume fats with carbohydrates in the same meal.

ABOUT THE WRITER: Vince Del Monte holds an Honors Kinesiology Degree and is a best-selling author. He's coined as the "Skinny Guy Savior" by over 80,000 former skinny men & women, who have followed his No Nonsense Muscle Building training and nutrition approach without drugs, bogus supplements, and in less time. Vince is also a *FitnessX Magazine* Cover Model. Contact Vince at www.VinceDelMonteFitness.com. Photo Credit: Noel Daganta

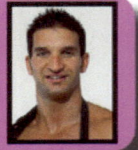

SECRETS TO LIVING AND FEELING HAPPY & HEALTHY

WRITTEN BY: Miranda Hoffmann

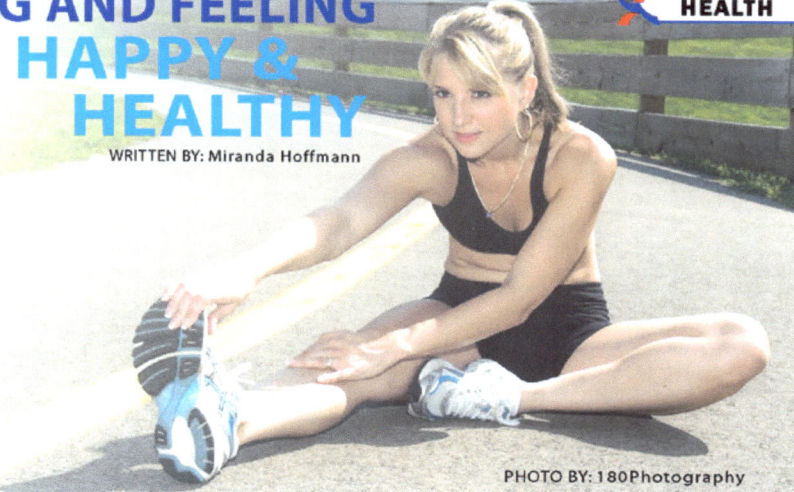

PHOTO BY: 180Photography

Everyone wants to feel happy and healthy, and BE happy and healthy. But what is the secret to getting there? There actually are a few ways to attain this, and they can be done every day.

1. Love yourself. Be happy with who you are. Feel comfortable being alone and spending time by yourself. Take the time to care for your body and your mind. Don't expect someone else to take care of you or make you happy…that's YOUR job. Love yourself enough to care for YOU. Love yourself enough to not let others HURT you. Love the person that you are and have respect for you.

2. Accept your mistakes and forgive yourself. This goes hand-in-hand with loving yourself. Understand that everyone makes mistakes and no one is perfect. Admit to yourself what your mistakes are. If possible, fix those mistakes. If you can't change them (because it's in the past), then accept that they happened and move on, learning from your mistake and not making the same mistake twice. Don't beat yourself up as this will not change anything. Love yourself enough to forgive yourself, and start over with your new knowledge. Understand that everyone will make many mistakes throughout their whole life and you are no exception. Worrying will never change the course of anything. But beating yourself up will bring you down faster than anything or anyone.

3. If you have trouble making decisions, flip a coin and be prepared to accept the consequences of the outcome, whichever it is. Don't waste precious time debating on a decision. If you absolutely, positively can't make a decision, then at that point it really doesn't make a difference what you choose. Apparently the pro's and con's of both are equivalent. Flip a coin, see what your answer is and stick to it. Deal with your decision. It's better than stressing over it day after day and never making a decision at all.

4. Accept others for who they are, don't stress yourself out by trying to change others. This is a biggie. I see more people holding on to a terrible amount of stress just from worrying about what someone else is doing or trying to change who they are. Stop bothering with other people and worry about yourself. You can give advice and try to help, but don't try to change someone. It never works and you will just end up losing sight of yourself. Besides, if you don't take care of yourself, how can you help someone else?

5. Look in the mirror and compliment yourself with beautiful words and inspiring affirmations. I know this may sound corny, but it works. When someone else feels bad, what do you do? You tell them nice things about them to make them feel better. What do you do for yourself when you feel bad? Beat yourself up. Not good. Don't wait on confirmation from others that you have good qualities. If you know it, tell yourself. Not sure what to say? There are websites and apps out there for free that will give or even send you an affirmation as often as you need it. Examples: 'I am truly blessed', 'I have unlimited choices in what I can think', 'I am a forgiving and loving person', 'I have unlimited potential, 'I deserve to be happy', 'I am talented', 'I deserve the very best in my life', 'I deserve love, success and happiness'. Compliment your positive attributes. You'd be amazed at how this will change your life. Suddenly you learn to respect yourself and stop belittling yourself. Most of the time we accept more pain and anguish from ourselves than we would ever allow from an outside source. The unfortunate part is that it's much more harmful.

6. Take care of your body. Yes, your body is your temple. If you don't care about your body and your health, then you don't care about YOU. Learn how to change bad habits. Hire help if you need it. Take pride in yourself. If you let your body waste away, what good are you to your friends and family? How can you achieve your goals if you are

sick, in the hospital, or worse yet, dead? Take your health seriuosly and CARE about YOU!

7. Eat every 2-3 hours. This is part of taking care of your body. Keep your blood sugar levels even. Get your metabolism pumped up and burn more calories at rest. Feel healthier. Make healthy choices. TAKE CARE OF YOURSELF. You only get one chance.

8. Busy? Take two 15 minute breaks each day….just for you. Allow yourself to enjoy the simple pleasures in life. What do you enjoy? Reading, painting, relaxing in front of the tv, talking to a friend on the phone? Pick something and take 15 minutes to enjoy those simple pleasures. You'll still get everything accomplished in your day as it is only a few minutes of your time, but it WILL do wonders for your brain and your soul.

9. Reward yourself by hiring someone to help you in your quest toward a better, happier life. You are not alone. Don't try to do it alone if you feel that you cannot. That's what we are here for! Personal trainers, life coaches, doctors, therapists…invest in your future. Start enjoying life!

10. Try to remind yourself that no matter how tough life gets, someone else out there has it harder. Count your blessings. Make a list of them if you need to and read it over whenever you feel overwhelmed. Many people have poor health, no family, no friends, no money… What do you have that you cherish? Focus on that during the hard times. Thank God for them and you'll find that when times are hard, you'll be able to deal with life a little better each time. Remember that a healthy body comes easier with a healthy, sound mind. Make yourself healthy from the inside out with positive thinking, healthy eating, and exercise. It's the "trifecta" of overall health! ✖

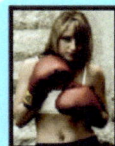

ABOUT THE WRITER: Miranda Hoffmann is a Certified Fitness Trainer through the International Sports Sciences Association (ISSA). She has been working as a fitness professional for over four years and takes pride in helping her clients achieve their goals. Her main focus is on weight loss, healthy weight gain, weight management, nutrition and lifestyle coaching, figure and bikini preparation and posing, and overall health. Whether in a gym setting, in-home training, or her corporate boot camps, you can be assured to get personal quality guidance and results.

Strength & Determination

Written By: Natalie Lynn Lichtenbert

When I was in my twenties, my late twenties that is, I was lucky enough to have a father that paid for my further education. He literally threw $1000 at me and said, "Go! Help yourself!" Before anything, make sure you work on your emotional health before even THINKING about going to the gym!

Believe it or not, I could be trusted with that money. I didn't spend it on going out. I didn't spend it on groceries. I didn't even spend it on clothes…and now for a girl such as myself, that might have been difficult! And to work through the negative things in life, build a positive attitude and to move forward, I had found it counter-productive to work with couselors and psychiatrists. Aside from being expensive, I felt I was re-hashing the old all the time or not focusing on the real issue. Let alone if you started seeing someone new, you'd have to start way back at the beginning…you never got anywhere!

So, being the introspective person that I am, I sought out literature that I could bring with me and read anytime of the day. For me, reading throughout the day, rather than waiting for the one-hour-a-week appointment, carried me much better to a happier outcome…that is, living a life of happiness, health and enjoyment. Along my journey, I read many of these books. I am going to share a few of them with you and how each one helped me along my journey!

One of the first books I bought out of my $1000 from my daddy was "Simple Abundance" by Sarah Ban Breathnach. This book literally has a passage to read for each day of the year. You could kind of say it became my little bible, having to read each day's message, usually a couple of pages long. "What is Self-Confidence?", "The Gift of Sacred Idleness" and "Answered Prayers" are just three of the topics to name a few. I will have to say, that although this book is written for women, I think it contains a lot of life lessons that all people could value from reading about. When I had bought it, I didn't start the book at

January either! The time of need help isn't always coming right at the beginning of a new year.

Book Two, "One Day My Soul Just Opened Up" by Iyanla Vanzant! Loved this one and still pick it up from time to time! I like this book because it

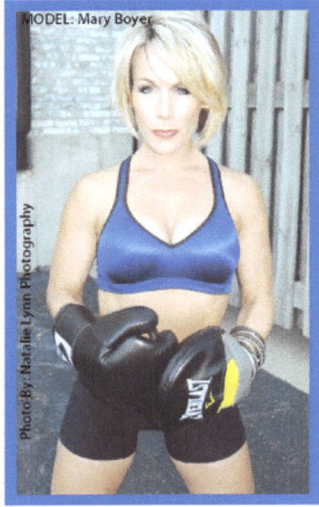

MODEL: Mary Boyer

Photo By: Natalie Lynn Photography

"I was now looking to create a life that contained new things like joy, laughter and accomplishment!"

goes through many of the emotions that we experience as people, her experiences and short stories relating to the emotion and then resolution. The

resolution involves things to keep in mind and exercises that help you to work through the emotion, for example anger or jealousy. To me, it is like a dictionary of emotions that you can look up at any time. This books helps you to understand how you are feeling, what is important to keep in mind at the time and how to move forward past the emotion…or to keep it in your life, for example, joy.

Well, by now I was starting to feel better, and Lord knows, there were certainly many other books along the way but one of the major ones to help me was called, "The Power of the Subconscious Mind" by Joseph Murphy, Ph.D, D.D. This book gave me my first insight to creating the life I wanted with my mind. I didn't realize how I was creating a life at that point by living in my past. I was now looking to create a life that contained new things like joy, laughter and accomplishment! It was by reading this book that I became aware of how to train my mind to rephrase those thoughts that were more negative into positive thoughts. Granted, old memories and scars can be hard to overcome, and most definitely can have a strong hold on you, but I was now starting to learn how to let go of those memories and thoughts and replacing them with good things.

Fourth and last book I will comment on, and am currently reading for the third (?) time is "The Secret" by Rhonda Byrne. I just love this book when it comes to really reaching up and grabbing all those things you ever wanted in your life! And I'm a believer!

Looking back, my life has never looked better! I'm excited to awake each day and to make each one special. Some days still have their challenges but they don't overwhelm me anymore, let alone get in between me and starting my day off in the gym! I continue to read, read, read and most certainly will have more books to share with you later…the growing never stops!

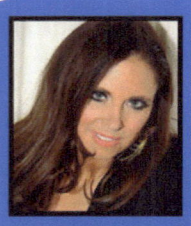

ABOUT THE WRITER: Born a dancer, Natalie Lynn Lichtenbert started her active career in ballet, tap, jazz, modern and hip hop dance styles. Also, being very active in sports, she participated in cheer, swimming and soccer. She currently keeps up her health and mental attitude while being a nationally recognized model, personal training, working as a photographer, continuing her fitness career, acting and following her environmental endeavors. She holds a Bachelor of Science in Medical Technology with extended studies in Molecular Pathology. She currently resides in Chicago, Illinois.

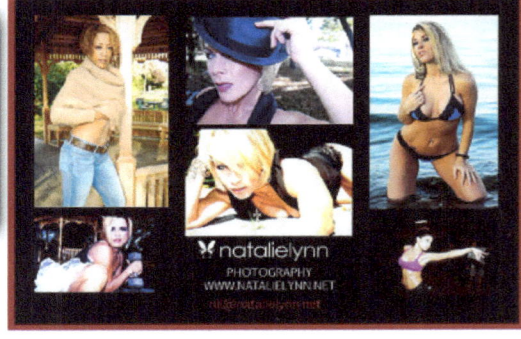

natalielynn
PHOTOGRAPHY
WWW.NATALIELYNN.NET

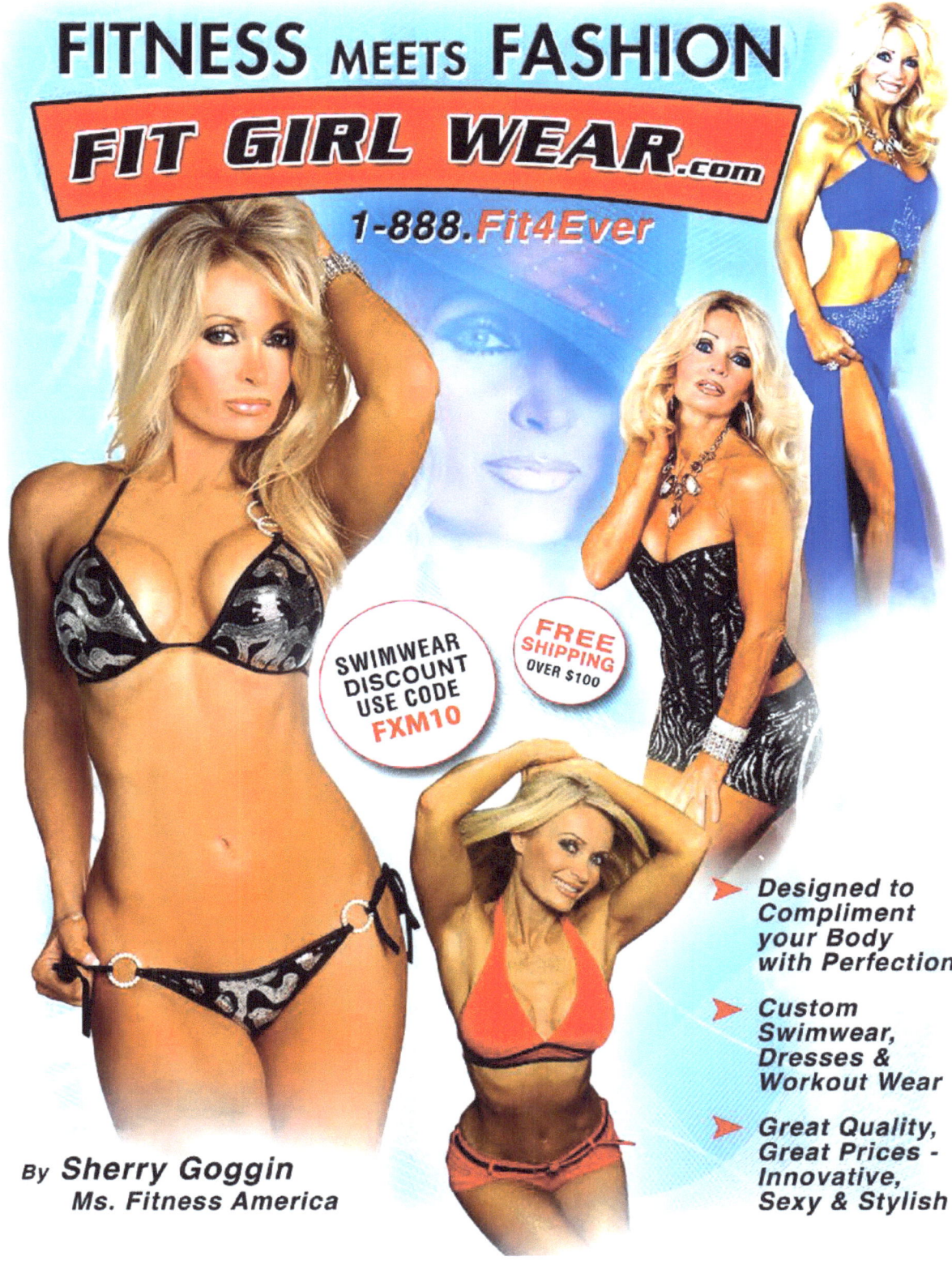